To Jack Christensen
Hey FB! Hope this will.
be a little help. Keep
on Stickin'!
Jack
Nick Seff.

Foreword

Seldom does a new book in a new subspecialty appear as fresh and as useful as this volume on oculoplastic surgery. It is a practical guide based on 30 years of extensive ophthalmic surgical practice combined with the teaching of techniques to residents. It has been kept simple and direct and, where possible, a point is often clarified by fine photographs and the superb drawings of Leon Schlossberg.

Dr. Charles E. Iliff, the senior author, is Professor of Ophthalmology at the Johns Hopkins University and School of Medicine. He is joined in this work by his two sons, Dr. W. Jackson Iliff and Dr. Nicholas T. Iliff, both in the private practice of ophthalmic surgery. All three attended Williams College, pursued their medical training at Johns Hopkins, and went through the Wilmer ophthalmological residency. The two younger authors have made invaluable contributions in helping to organize much of the text to make it more useful to the less experienced surgeon, without dulling its interest or importance as an atlas for the more difficult procedures.

The book is a masterpiece and will be enjoyed by the neophyte and master surgeon alike.

WENDELL L. HUGHES, M.D., F.A.C.S., D.Sc.

Preface

A new subspecialty—ophthalmic reconstructive surgery—has emerged. It seems timely, therefore, to gather together in one volume techniques that have been successful in our hands through the years and to present them in a manner that could be helpful to those whose interests bring them to this field.

No claims are made to originality, nor is this book a review of the literature. Rather, the procedures presented in this volume are based on the senior author's 30 years of experience. The operations have been adopted, with successful results, by a second generation of oculoplastic surgeons in this family. In developing the manuscript we have worked and re-worked the text to make the surgical procedures understandable to the senior surgeon, the young practicing surgeon, and the house officer alike. To clarify points in the text, the procedures are illustrated step-by-step and further elucidated by the drawings of Leon Schlossberg. This book is meant to be a working manual of operations as practiced by the authors.

Sincere appreciation and acknowledgment must be attributed to our teachers and colleagues, Wendell L. Hughes, Edmund B. Spaeth, Crowell Beard, Raynold Berke, Sydney A. Fox, Alston Callahan, John C. Mustardé, Byron Smith, Lester Jones, and others, who have contributed their thoughts by word or writing.

David Andrews reviewed our work and made suggestions for the organization and presentation of this material, and Dorothy Louey typed and retyped the manuscript until her knowledge of the subject rivals that of any of the authors. For their devoted help, we are very grateful.

CHARLES E. ILIFF, M.D.
W. JACKSON ILIFF, M.D.
NICHOLAS T. ILIFF, M.D.

Contents

1
Surgical Principles

Ophthalmic plastic surgery differs from general plastic surgery primarily because of the extraordinary qualities of the skin of the lids. The techniques of suturing, grafting, and reconstruction using skin flaps are dictated by skin pliability, softness, thinness, and vascularity unmatched elsewhere in the body. Although these qualities may make some reconstructive maneuvers more feasible, the narrow margin between successful and unsuccessful functional result makes ophthalmic plastic surgery most challenging.

Instrumentation

The absolute need to minimize scarring if function is to be maintained or restored requires a totally atraumatic approach. It goes without saying that the instruments, sutures, and needles used should be as fine in construction as possible. It is often necessary to handle flaps of tissue no more than 2 or 3 mm wide; such tissue is easily disrupted by careless manipulation with overly stout forceps and can be easily strangled by a large or improperly placed suture. Skin of the lids should, when at all possible, be handled with fine skin hooks to preclude any crushing effect. Should forceps be needed, 0.3 mm toothed forceps are usually adequate; however, 0.12 mm forceps may be appropriate for the handling of the more friable tissues.

Sharp-pointed spring action straight iris scissors have proved to be the best instrument when fine, sharp dissection is needed. Conventional scissors without spring action and with larger blades can be cumbersome. The pliability and laxness of lid skin make accurate incision with a scalpel difficult. A more satisfactory approach is to make lid skin incisions entirely with sharp iris scissors or to mark the proposed incision line with a very light scalpel touch and complete the incision with scissors. In this way, bunching of the skin, with subsequent distortion of the anatomy, is avoided.

In ophthalmic plastic surgery, the success of an operation often depends on accurate identification of structures as they are dissected. Blind or undue dissection of a lid can cause failure. Hemorrhage must be controlled at all times to permit ready visualization of structures. Time is rarely a factor, and meticulous dry dissection is always essential. This cannot be done without hemostasis; therefore, the necessary time should be taken to keep the field dry. Postoperative hematoma can cause a graft to fail or can cause scarring with secondary loss of some lid function. In the extreme case, eyesight can be lost. Hemostasis at the time of operation cannot be overstressed. Anesthetic agents containing vasoconstrictors are helpful in prolonging anesthesia and keeping a dry field. It must be remembered, however, that vasoconstrictors can give the surgeon a false sense of security. A seemingly dry field at close may occasionally give rise to postoperative hemorrhage when the effects of vasoconstriction are gone. Cautery should not be limited, but it should not be used indiscriminately. It is best to identify and cauterize each bleeding point as it appears. If there is diffuse bleeding or bleeding from a site that cannot be seen, pressure can be used to control it. Postoperative dressings should be designed to apply the appropriate pressure to the operative site without endangering the circulation of the eye. During the operative procedure, diffuse bleeding may be temporarily controlled with the application of a topical vasoconstrictor (phenylephrine, adrenalin). Recently, collagen materials (Avitene) have been used successfully to control bleeding.

Suturing Technique

The skin of the lid is the thinnest of the body and requires some aspects of suturing technique not necessary elsewhere. All suturing techniques can be used, but some are more suitable than others.

Both interrupted and running stitches can be used — each type has its own advantages. When fine absorbable sutures are being used deep in the lid, interrupted sutures have several advantages: (1) The kind of distortion of tissue planes caused by bunching along a running suture is eliminated. (2) Control of individual stitch tension is possible. (3) If one suture breaks, the entire suture line is not disrupted. However, when the levator aponeurosis and conjunctiva are being sutured in ptosis operations, running sutures are advantageous. They provide a flat suture and only one or two knots (minimizing the threat of corneal abrasion); the tarsal plate provides a firm structure to prevent distortion.

Interrupted sutures have, likewise, proved to be the best method for skin closure. Individual stitch tension can more easily be controlled. Taking a minute bite of epithelium at each skin edge and tying the stitch slightly tighter than would be done elsewhere allows the suture to fall out in four to five days in most instances and does not leave a suture mark. Distortion of the wound is difficult to avoid if a continuous suture is used on the lax skin of the lid. Single arm suturing is used for most skin incision closures. A fine bite with very thin suture material minimizes scarring. It is always important to evert skin edges. In some cases, the incision may be under mild tension, particularly if it extends into the thicker skin at the temple, cheek, or brow. A vertical mattress suture provides more strength and allows for fine approximation of the skin edges. It is important to take out these sutures in three to five days, for although suture marks are extremely rare in the skin of the lid, they can occur in the thicker surrounding skin.

Whether or not suture marks occur depends on several factors. Most important is the length of time the sutures are left in. Suture marks can occur adjacent to the eyelids if sutures are left in ten days or more; they rarely occur if sutures are taken out before one week. The distance sutures are placed from the wound edges is important; the closer to the edge, the less likely it is that a mark will be formed. Because of their distance from the wound edge, vertical mattress sutures should not be left in for extended periods. Excessive suture tension and infection also contribute to the formation of suture marks.

Horizontal mattress sutures are useful for everting skin edges. They are used primarily at the lid margins for tarsorrhaphy or in lid splitting procedures done for reconstruction purposes.

Subcuticular sutures (sutures passed through the dermis in a continuous fashion) give a very nice closure with minimal scarring but are difficult to do well on the extremely thin skin of the lid and offer no advantages over interrupted skin sutures.

Two or three layer closure can be important to minimize dead space where blood or serous fluid can collect or infection can start. In addition, closure of deep layers is important to support the skin and relieve tension on the incision. Tension on an incision can cause widening of a scar or breakdown of the suture line.

Routine skin closure is done with 8–0 black silk on an atraumatic needle. If more strength is needed (as at the canthi or on the cheek or brow), 7–0 or 6–0 can be used, but in general the smaller the better. If there is no tension on the incision, it can be closed with 8–0. Silk is easier to manage than nylon, is less irritating should a suture end come in contact with the globe, can be tied easily, and suture tension is more easily controlled. In larger sizes, Ethiflex or other synthetic braided sutures can be used, but they have no real advantage over silk. Absorbable suture for skin closure has a place in surgery on children because it eliminates the need for removal. 7–0 is the best choice, and catgut works as well as synthetic absorbables. However, the added inflammation caused by absorbable sutures is better avoided if the possibility of easy suture removal makes the use of silk sutures practical.

Scars

As has been mentioned, avoidance of scarring is the ideal of functional and cosmetic ophthalmic plastic surgery. Scars cannot be

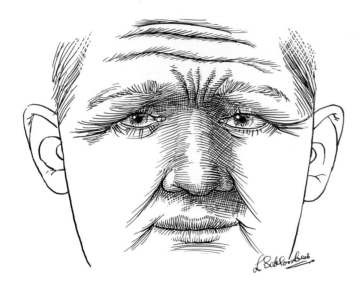

Figure 1–1 Distribution of useful wrinkles.

avoided; they can only be minimized. One of the important ways of minimizing a scar is to cause it to fall in a pre-existing wrinkle or crease (Fig. 1–1). The majority of facial wrinkles are formed by a slight infolding of skin perpendicular to the axis of contraction of an underlying muscle. Placing an incision closure in one of the many wrinkles available will minimize interference with function and help achieve the best possible appearance.

Scars contract equally per unit breadth or length as they evolve. Therefore a scar 0.5 mm wide and 1 cm long will contract 20 times as much along its longitudinal axis as it will perpendicular to that axis. This contraction should always be kept in mind because it can cause hooding following blepharoplasty (Fig. 1–2), or ectropion or notching of the lower lid if incision or laceration is perpendicular to the lid margin. Incisions should be oriented so that this longitudinal contraction either occurs in the least harmful direction or is minimized in one direction by some form of "Z" or "W" incision. Gentle handling of skin edges, avoidance of hemorrhage or infection,

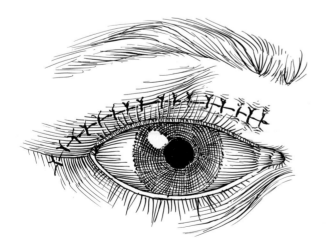 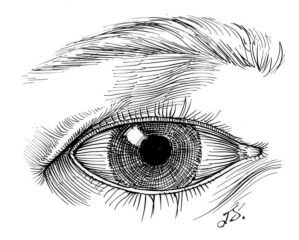

Figure 1–2 Hooding caused by contraction of the scar from an incision carried around the canthus.

prevention of inversion of skin edges, minimizing of wound tension, as accomplished by suturing of deep layers and undermining, and proper suture tension are all factors in minimizing scars at operation. Postoperatively, certain measures can be taken to further minimize scarring. Application of a bland ointment in the early postoperative days is helpful in keeping wound edges soft and promoting good union. Use of ointment at the time of operation is not advisable because it may get between the skin margins and inhibit primary union. The normal evolution of a scar is from a mildly raised pinkish ridge (more prominent in children) to a flat white line. The firmness of the ultimate scar can often be altered significantly by softening creams and massage. Mild postoperative cicatricial ectropion or lagophthalmos frequently can be eliminated by digital massage with skin cream several times a day.

The most important inhibitor of damaging scar formation is the nature of the skin of the lid. The extremely thin, pliable, dermis-poor skin of the lid forms almost no scars. In general, the thicker the dermis, the more scar skin will form in a particular location. It is imperative for the best result to confine incisions and reconstructive maneuvers to the lids themselves. Incisions into the thicker skin of the nose, cheek, or brow should be avoided whenever possible. Blowout fractures, for instance, should be approached through an incision in the lid skin followed by dissection down to the orbital rim rather than through the thicker skin at the orbital rim where an unsightly scar is certain. Likewise, a dacryocystorhinostomy can easily be done through the normal lid crease over the lacrimal crest and need not be approached through the thicker, more scar-prone skin of the nose, as is advocated by many surgeons.

Skin Grafting

Loss of tissue of the lids as a result of trauma, tumor removal, or overzealous cosmetic surgery can cause distressing functional and cosmetic damage. Replacement can be carried out through skin grafting from a distal donor site or through relocation of adjacent tissues to minimize or eliminate a defect. Skin grafting to the lid has more stringent requirements than skin grafting to any other part of the body. The primary difficulty is obtaining skin that is thin enough and pliable enough to be used on the lid. The upper lid has the strictest limits in this regard; the use of slightly less pliable skin is possible in the lower lid. In addition, as with any skin graft to the face, texture and color match are essential if cosmetic acceptance is to be achieved.

Skin grafts are of two major types — split thickness and full thickness. A split thickness graft consists of the epidermis and a portion of the dermis. Split thickness grafts can be considered thin, intermediate, or thick, depending on the depth of the cut that is made into the dermis at the donor site (as determined by the setting of the dermatome — .010 to .025 inch), the translucency of the graft, and the bleeding at the donor site (Fig. 1–3). A thin graft is

agreeable color match. The supraclavicular area is a good donor site for split or full thickness grafts. Color and texture match are nearly as good as for the postauricular area, and large donor pieces can be obtained. However, women often object to this site because the resulting scar lies in a frequently exposed area.

Preputial skin provides an excellent match for upper lid skin if relatively large amounts of extremely pliable donor skin are needed. However, not only is this not often available, but the usual hyperpigmentation causes a poor color match. The inner thigh can be used if no other donor areas are available (for instance, as a result of extensive burns). A split thickness graft must be taken. The graft tends to become yellowish or brown, and the thinner the graft, the browner it may become. Other donor sites include the abdomen, the inner upper arm, and the upper lateral chest wall (particularly in women). Each of these can provide split thickness grafts but are tertiary choices for replacement of lid skin.

THE RECIPIENT BED

Lids and periocular tissues are highly vascular, making skin grafting in this area very successful and, therefore, useful. Graft survival is the rule rather than the exception because an excellent nutrient bed is usually available. However, heavily irradiated tissue is a relatively poor recipient bed because of its poor blood supply. Bone denuded of periosteum in general will not support a skin graft; however, a bare orbit can be lined with a split thickness graft and it will survive without problem (see Exenteration in Chapter 9).

SURVIVAL OF SKIN GRAFTS

During the initial 48 hours after grafting, a plasma-like fluid is absorbed into the graft. Some red blood cells are drawn in with this fluid. Only the deeper portions of the graft can be nourished in this way. This in part contributes to the superior viability of a thin graft versus a thick one. Subsequently, a vascular circulation in the graft is re-established, initially by the anastamosis of bed vessels with the deeper vessels of the graft by way of vascular channels established in the fibrin network that binds the skin graft to its recipient site.*

The tertiary event is the ingrowth of new capillaries and then establishment of lymphatic drainage.†

PREPARATION OF THE GRAFT

Skin from an upper lid, after being carefully excised with sharp-pointed scissors, can be sutured into place with no further

*Clemmesen, T.: The early circulation in split-skin grafts. Restoration of blood supply to split-skin autografts. *Acta Chir. Scand.,* 127:1, 1964, and Smith, J. W., Ringland, J., and Wilson, R.: Vascularization of skin grafts. *Surg. Forum,* 15:473, 1964.

†Converse, J. M., and Ballantyne, D. L., Jr.: Distribution of diphosphorpyridine nucleotide diaphorase in rat skin autografts and homografts. *Plast. Reconstr. Surg.,* 30:415, 1962.

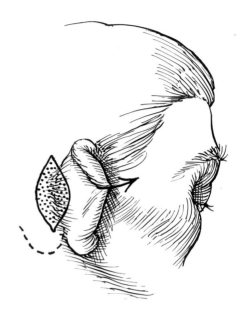

Figure 1–4   Postauricular graft.

preparation. Take only as much skin from the donor lid as can be taken with the eye closed. Postauricular skin is removed from the pinna and temporal area (Fig. 1–4) in an elliptical fashion, leaving an incision which can be closed primarily. Full thickness supraclavicular grafts should be cut in elliptical fashion for easy closure. These, like those from the postauricular area, may need some trimming of the subcutaneous tissue and fat to leave only epidermis and dermis. The thinnest possible graft is obtained by pinning the graft on a small board (25-gauge, 5/8 inch hypodermic needles are handy for this) and cutting away the excess tissue with the curved aspect of fine spring action scissors. The graft is cut to the approximate proper shape, and the remainder of the shaping is done after the graft is partially sutured in place. This procedure assures a good fit and allows for proper tension. Careful suture of the graft margin with 8–0 black silk produces minimal scarring.

A split thickness graft can be taken from the supraclavicular area by ballooning up the skin with 100 to 200 cc of saline. The injection sites must be outside the limits of the graft so that leakage from the needle holes will not interfere with the cutting of the graft. For work around the eye, grafts from the arm, abdomen, or leg are usually split thickness. The donor site is prepared in the usual fashion. A Stryker adhesive sheet is applied to the area. The dermatome (Stryker) is set at .010 to .015 inch and used to cut the graft. (The Stryker dermatome is calibrated to account for the thickness of the adhesive sheet — thus a graft of .010 to .015 inch is obtained.) A firm pressure is maintained while the assistant helps extract the graft, adherent to the plastic sheet, as it emerges from the dermatome. The donor site is dressed with a nonadherent dressing (Telfa, Xeroform) and a pressure dressing. The graft should be kept moist until it is placed on the recipient bed.

Good contact between the graft and recipient bed is essential for survival of the graft. A clot or collection of serous fluid must be evacuated or vascularization will be delayed and autolysis will set in. Improper tension can prevent proper apposition of the graft to the bed. If too loose, wrinkles will form and leave some areas out of contact. A tight graft will bridge depressions in the bed rather than follow them. Careful hemostasis is essential, followed by a moderate pressure dressing to prevent later accumulation of blood or serous fluid. Several small drainage holes in the graft are helpful in allowing fluid to escape. The graft should be inspected by at least the second postoperative day and any fluid drained. Repeated drainage of serous fluid or blood may be necessary to assure contact between graft and bed.

Tie-over dressings in which half the suture ends are left long and tied over a bulky dressing placed over the graft are excellent for immobilizing a small graft. However, we have rarely found this type of dressing necessary. A dressing carefully applied with tape can take care of most situations. A removable dressing allows inspection of the graft at 48 hours, after which the patient is discharged from the hospital. With the very thin grafts of the lids and adjacent areas, immobilization for approximately two to five days is adequate. However, excessive motion or manipulation of the graft — even so slight as the changing of the dressing — can cause shearing between the graft and bed with a loss of the nutrition channels to the graft and possibly the production of a seroma or hematoma.

Mucous Membrane Grafts

Mucous membrane grafts are frequently needed for lid or cul-de-sac reconstruction. The primary donor sites are the inner lower lip or cheek. The use of nasal mucous membrane is described; however, we have felt its use unnecessary. The Castroviejo mucotome has not worked well in our hands, and we have therefore preferred to use thin full thickness grafts cut in a free-hand manner. The lower lip is everted and stretched over a large lip clamp. A scalpel is used to very lightly outline the borders of the graft. Blunt-pointed (Wescott) scissors are then used to carefully dissect under the graft. Dissection is facilitated by leaving the graft margins attached until the undermining is completed. After the graft is freed, a gauze pack is put between the lip and the teeth and the lip is allowed to return to its normal position. No suturing is necessary because the open bed will completely epithelialize in about a week. The patient should avoid solid or crumbly foods for 72 hours postoperatively. Even when large grafts (2 × 4 cm) have been taken, patients rarely have had significant discomfort.

The newly cut graft is pinned on a small board, and the fat and connective tissue adherent to the undersurface are removed as is done with a full thickness skin graft. Very thin mucous membrane grafts can be obtained in this free-hand fashion, but great care must be taken in their preparation. The graft is sutured in place with interrupted 8–0 or 7–0 absorbable sutures with the knots buried. Any suturing of conjunctiva or mucous membrane on the globe or inner surface of the lid should be done with buried knots to avoid patient discomfort and the possibility of corneal abrasion.

Skin Flaps

Skin flaps are extremely useful for lid and periorbital reconstructions. The thin skin of the lid is amenable to a variety of flap types that are less feasible in other areas. Skin flaps in general tend to be bulky and thick. However, the types used around the eye usually are quite delicate owing to their size and the thinness of the skin. The superb vascularity of the area allows the use of flap shapes that would not survive elsewhere. However, the surgeon should consider skin grafts first, for they are easier to do and may give as good results cosmetically as skin flaps.

The most frequently used types of local skin flaps are (1) bilobed; (2) pedicle — advancement and rotation, (3) V–Y, and (4) Z-plasty. In all cases, careful planning is essential before incisions are made.

Bilobed Flaps. The bilobed flap allows the surgeon to fill the primary defect with a flap and then transpose a second flap from an area of more lax tissue to fill the secondary defect left by the primary flap (Fig. 1–5).

Pedicle Flaps. The advancement or sliding flap is a rectangular or square flap of skin and subcutaneous tissue that takes advantage of the elasticity of the skin. At the base of the flap, triangular excisions (Bürow's triangles) help to equalize the length between sides of the flap and the adjacent wound margins (Fig. 1–6). These flaps are particularly valuable in reconstruction of lower lids following excision of tumors. It is important to orient the flap horizontally rather than vertically, for vertical tension on the lid can result in ectropion.

Another type of pedicle flap is one that is rotated about an axis at its base. In general, pedicle flaps cannot be more than two to three times as long as they are wide or the distal aspect of the flap will not survive owing to poor vascular supply. However, this applies to thick flaps that rely heavily on the vessels passing through the pedicle. Pedicle flaps in oculoplastic surgery are of great help in moving skin from one portion of a lid to another or from a lid to an adjacent lid. Since the skin of the lid is so thin and has minimal

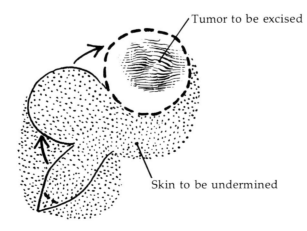
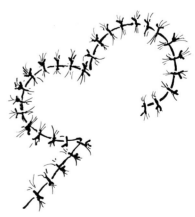

Figure 1–5 Bilobed flap.

Tumor to be excised

Skin to be undermined

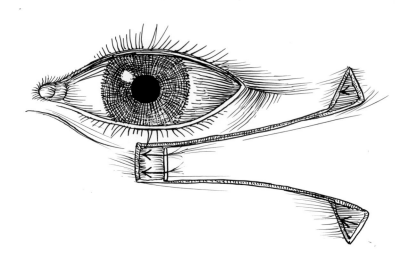

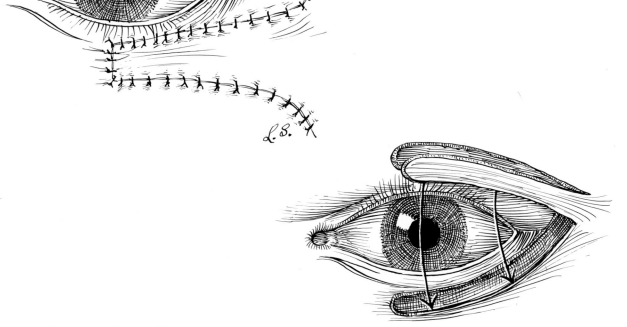

Figure 1–6 Advancement flap.

Figure 1–7 Pedicle flap.

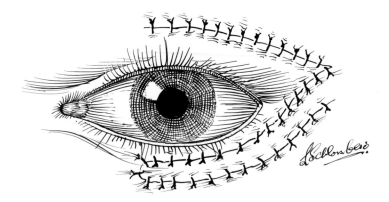

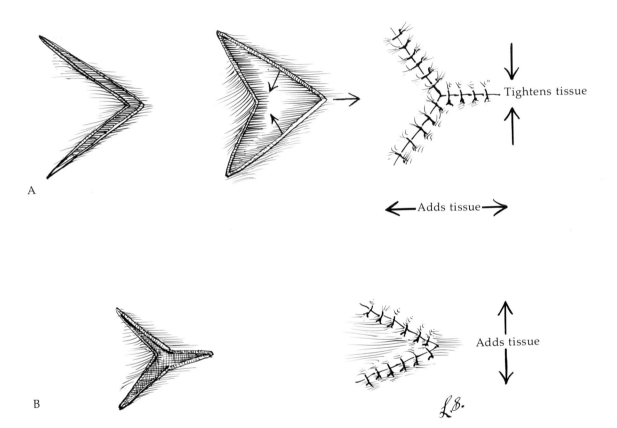

Figure 1–8 Advancement technique. *A,* V–Y. *B,* Y–V.

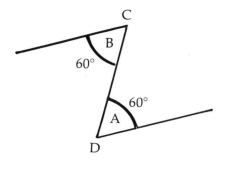 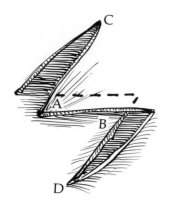 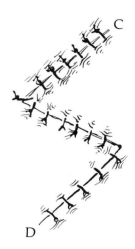

Figure 1–9   Z-plasty.

subcutaneous tissue, the flap acts as a free skin graft that has the added advantage of an already vascularized pedicle. As a result, a length to width ratio of 5 to 1 is easily used when lid skin only is being transferred (Fig. 1–7). Rarely do these flaps fail to survive.

V–Y Flaps.   To close the donor site of a skin flap, to relieve tension on the lid margin, or to ease the effect of a tight scar or band of skin, a V–Y advancement technique can be used. A V-shaped incision can be closed to a "Y," thus adding more tissue in the long axis of the "Y" while decreasing it perpendicular to the axis (Fig. 1–8*A*). Likewise, if a Y-shaped incision has been made and there is tension perpendicular to it, the skin at the top of the "Y" can be advanced and closed as a "V" (Fig. 1–8*B*).

Z-Plasty Flaps.   The Z-plasty consists of the interchanging of two triangular flaps. The procedure is done to increase the length of tissue in a desired direction, to break the continuity of a long scar or realign it, or to transpose the tissue included in the Z-plasty flap (e.g., the eyebrow). The arms of the "Z" must be equal in length to the central member. The angle between the arms and the center of the "Z" can vary from 30 to 90 degrees, but angles greater than 60 degrees are technically difficult and rarely useful (Fig. 1–9). The greater the angle, the greater is the percentage gain in length along the axis of the central member; the longer the central member, the greater will be the actual gain in length.

Z-plasty flaps can be used in several ways:

1. Tissue along the scar contraction (Fig. 1–10) can be lengthened by aligning the central member of the "Z" to lie on the scar (with excision of scar if necessary).
2. Occasionally a scar can be realigned to fall in a natural skin fold; however, more often a scar can be made less conspicuous by interrupting its continuity by multiple small Z-plasties.
3. Z-plasties are helpful for the rotation of the tissue contained in the flaps. Malpositioned lateral canthus or eyebrow can occasionally be elevated or lowered with a simple Z-plasty for significant cosmetic improvement (Fig. 1–11).

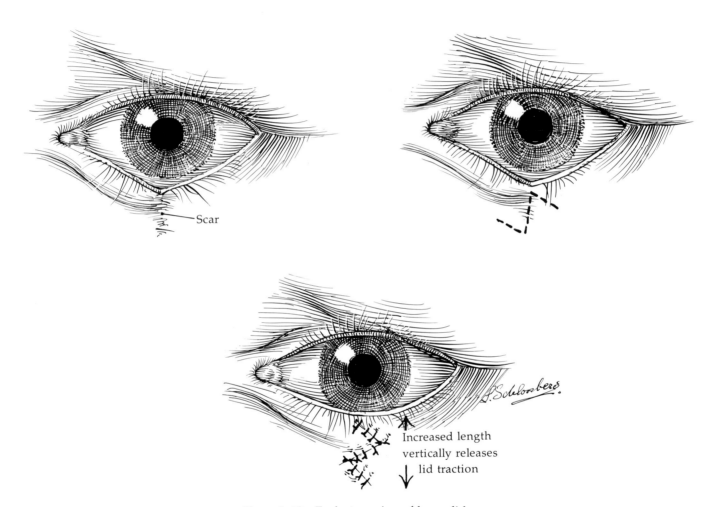

Figure 1–10   Z-plasty easing of lower lid scar.

Scar

Increased length
vertically releases
lid traction

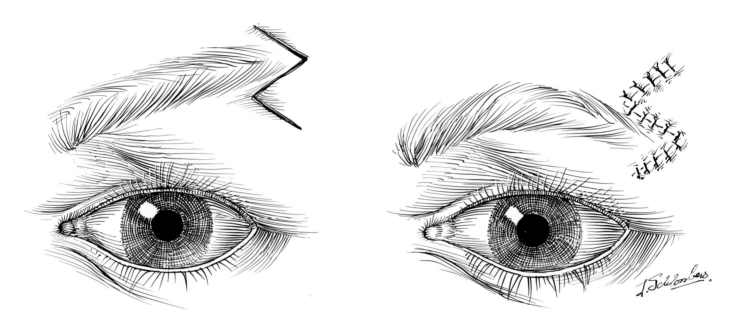

Figure 1–11   Brow Z-plasty.

SKIN FLAP TECHNIQUE

In all cases, flaps, like skin grafts, should be handled with the utmost care. Fine (8–0) single armed sutures are used to close the incisions, with special care being taken to avoid strangulating the tentative vascular supply to the flap tip. Careful hemostasis to the bed, with minimal but effective cautery to the flap, is important. A mild pressure dressing is used. Following the first dressing change, ointment should be applied to keep the skin graft or flap (particularly at its poorly vascularized margins) from drying.

Because of the excellent vascularity already mentioned, it is rare for a skin flap to fail if it consists only of the skin of and around the eyelids. However, should ischemia or infection cause failure of the flap, the area should be allowed to heal and—if necessary—the resulting scar can be excised and replaced with a skin graft.

2

Ptosis

The goal of ptosis surgery is to raise the lid above the visual axis and to create as perfect a cosmetic result as possible by attaining symmetry of the lid height, lid folds, and lid motion. Thus both static and dynamic symmetry are sought. With the eye in the primary position, the upper lid normally crosses the cornea 1.5 to 2.0 mm below the superior limbus, and the lid crease is just above the retrotarsal margin (Fig. 2–1). These are static consider-

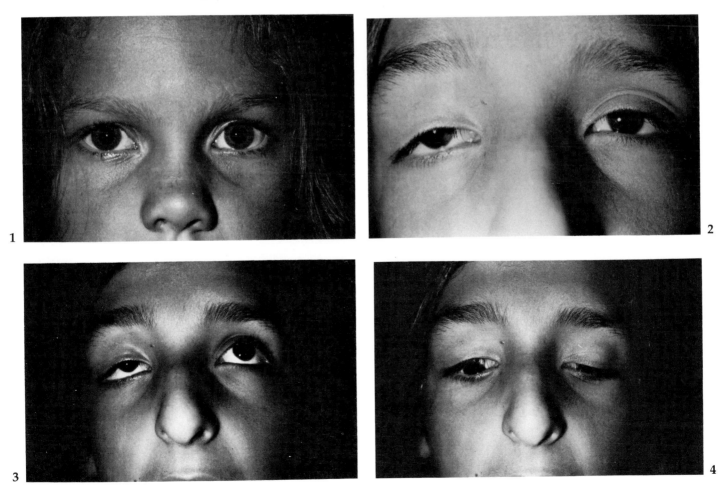

Figure 2–1 Normal lid contour and position.
Figures 2–2, 2–3, 2–4 Congenital ptosis.

ations. As the eye moves upward and downward, the normal lid follows the globe and maintains its position just below the superior limbus. These are the dynamic considerations.

A ptosed lid crosses the cornea at a point more than 2 mm below the upper limbus and usually is limited in its range of motion or in its ability to follow the globe in elevation and often in depression (Figs. 2–2 to 2–4). Two acceptable surgical approaches have been developed to correct these defects. The action of the primary elevators of the lid, the levator muscle and Mueller's muscle, can be increased, or if this is not possible, a secondary elevator of the lid (the frontalis muscle) can be utilized.

SURGICAL ANATOMY OF THE UPPER LID

SKIN

The skin of the lids is extremely thin, loose, and mobile over the orbicularis muscle, as far as the brow above, where it joins the thicker skin of the forehead, and the orbital rim below, where it joins the skin of the cheek. The histological junction between skin and conjunctiva is located just posterior to the openings of the meibomian gland ducts, but for surgical purposes the skin of the lid terminates at the gray line. An important surgical landmark, the gray line is a lightly pigmented line at the lid margin that separates the skin-muscle layer anteriorly from the tarsal-conjunctival layer posteriorly. The extreme thinness of the skin of the lid (0.6 mm average) is essential to normal lid function and appearance. In young persons the lid skin is quite elastic but with aging the normal elasticity is lost, the dermis thins, and the skin becomes redundant.

The eyelashes (cilia) are arranged in two or three irregular rows at the anterior aspect of the lid margins. In the upper lid, after emerging from the lids in a slightly downward direction, they curve upward. The reverse is true in the lower lid. The skin of the lid has other very fine hairs, which often are hard to see. The ducts of eccrine sweat glands empty onto the skin. The holocrine sebaceous glands (the glands of Zeis) empty into the lash follicles. The glands of Moll are apocrine sweat glands that also empty into the lash follicles.

ORBICULARIS MUSCLE

Beneath the skin and the thin subcutaneous matrix is the orbicularis muscle, which closes the lid. That it is much stronger than the retractor muscles that open the lids becomes apparent if one tries to force open the lids of an uncooperative baby. On the other hand, a lid can be held closed with a very slight pressure of the finger. The orbicularis muscle is divided into the pretarsal and preseptal portions, with fibers coursing in a horizontal elliptical direction across and around the lids to join at the medial and lateral canthal tendons. Fibers from the levator aponeurosis and orbital septum penetrate the orbicularis muscle at the upper level of the tarsus to insert in the subcutaneous tissue and skin, producing the lid crease. The orbicularis muscle fibers are striated and receive their innervation from the seventh cranial nerve.

FRONTALIS MUSCLE

The frontalis muscle originates from the galea aponeurotica above the hairline and inserts into the deep skin of the brows. It is a secondary elevator of the lid, transmitting its pull through the skin, subcutaneous tissue, and orbital septum to the lid. The excursion of the muscle is the greatest at the orbital rim, as can be demonstrated by placing the finger along the cilia of the brow and contracting the muscle. It is supplied by the seventh cranial nerve.

ORBITAL SEPTUM

The orbital septum lies posterior to the orbicularis muscle. It is a thin sheet of fibrous tissue that originates from the periosteum of the superior orbital rim and hangs down like a curtain across the entire lid to join, by interdigitating fibers, with the levator aponeurosis at approximately the level of the upper edge of the tarsus. Joined, the orbital septum and levator aponeurosis pass downward to insert on the lower anterior surface of the tarsus. The septum spreads nasally to the posterior lacrimal crest and temporally to the fascia of the lacrimal gland. The septum can be identified by placing a finger just beneath the orbital rim and putting traction on the lid margin. This tension on the orbital septum can be felt as it is transmitted to the brow.

ORBITAL FAT

The orbital fat lies behind the septum and is a lobulated, loosely supported structure containing many fine small blood vessels and nerves. There are numerous membranous septae dividing the lobules. The fat is quite thin at the retrotarsal margin and thickens in a wedge formation as it passes back into the orbit. It is an important surgical landmark, as it separates the orbital septum from the levator aponeurosis and muscle; the orbital septum lies anterior to, and the levator aponeurosis posterior to, the fat pocket.

LEVATOR MUSCLE

The levator muscle is a primary elevator of the lid; its failure to function properly produces a ptosis. It originates from the periorbita just above the annulus of Zinn and passes forward above the superior rectus muscle and beneath the frontal nerve. It is narrow at its origin and gradually widens as it extends anteriorly, until it blends into its tendon. The tendon fans out to form the aponeurosis, which is the full width of the lid at the upper level of the tarsus. Here the tendon fuses with the orbital septum and together they pass forward to insert in the anterior lower third of the tarsus

darker in color than the levator muscle, and firmly adherent to the conjunctiva just posterior to it. For these reasons, few surgeons are able to isolate it as a distinct entity at the time of operation.

WHITNALL'S LIGAMENT

Whitnall's ligament (the superior transverse ligament) is a condensation of the levator sheath. The ligament in most instances is anterior to the levator, but sometimes it surrounds it like an envelope. Extending laterally to the orbital lobe of the lacrimal gland and nasally to the fascia of the trochlea, this ligament, like the horns, may act as a check on the levator muscle, restricting its motion.

LACRIMAL GLAND

The lacrimal gland is composed of two lobes, an anterior palpebral lobe and a posterior orbital lobe. These lie in the lacrimal fossa of the upper temporal portion of the bony orbit. The lateral horn of the levator aponeurosis passes between the anterior and posterior lobes and on to the fascia of the lateral canthal ligament. The secreting ducts of the orbital lobe of the lacrimal gland pass around the edge of the levator aponeurosis, through the palpebral lobe, and join with the palpebral lobe ducts to empty into the lateral aspect of the superior conjunctival fornix.

Tears secreted from the gland pass from the ducts into the upper lateral cul-de-sac and sweep across the cornea to empty into the lacrimal drainage system.

SUPERIOR RECTUS MUSCLE

The superior rectus muscle, which is innervated by the third cranial nerve, lies beneath the levator; both the levator and superior rectus muscle send small branches of fascia to the conjunctiva of the upper cul-de-sac. When the eye is rotated upward, these fibers pull the conjunctiva of the fornix upward and backward to move with the lid and the globe.

THE TARSUS

The tarsus, the skeleton of the upper lid, is a fibrous plate about 1 mm thick with a horizontal dimension of 22 to 25 mm and a vertical dimension of 8 to 9 mm. It contains the meibomian glands, which secrete lipid from their openings along the inferior margin of the lid. The levator aponeurosis, with the associated orbital septum, attaches to the anterior inferior one third of the tarsus. Mueller's muscle attaches to the retrotarsal margin. As the levator muscle contracts, the tarsus is pulled upward and backward and the relatively free retrotarsal margin closely follows the globe.

THE CONJUNCTIVA

The conjunctiva is firmly attached to the posterior aspect of the tarsus. This mucous membrane contains numerous mucin-secreting goblet cells, concentrated primarily in the fornices. It covers the tarsus and Mueller's muscle and then reflects on itself in the upper fornix to extend down over the globe as far as the limbus. At the upper fornix, the fine connective tissue fibers from both the levator and the superior rectus muscle insert into the conjunctiva to pull the fornix upward and backward as the eye and lid are elevated. The ducts of the lacrimal gland pass through the conjunctiva to empty into the upper temporal fornix. The accessory lacrimal glands of Wolfring and Krause are supported by the palpebral conjunctiva. The conjunctiva passes around the tarsal edge at the lid margin to join the skin just posterior to the openings of the meibomian glands.

VASCULAR SUPPLY

The two main arteries to the upper lid lie in the pretarsal space. The marginal arcade runs along the edge of the lids and the peripheral arcade branches from the marginal arcade and runs along the upper part of the tarsus. These arcades are fed temporally by the zygomatic orbital artery from the facial and external carotid arteries and nasally from the angular artery (a branch of the internal carotid). The veins of the lids have an erratic pattern but drain into the ophthalmic, the angular, and the temporal veins. The vascularity of the lid is extensive, promoting rapid healing of the lid following trauma and surgery, but also at times causing difficulties during surgery.

Summary

The skin of the lid is the thinnest and softest skin of the body. Beneath the loose subcutaneous tissue lies the orbicularis muscle, responsible for the forceful closing of the lids. The orbital septum lies deep to the orbicularis and extends from the periosteum of the brow to insert along with the levator aponeurosis in the anterior inferior aspect of the tarsus. Orbital fat, an important and easily recognizable landmark of the lid, lies between the orbital septum and levator aponeurosis above the point where these two structures join. The levator is a much weaker muscle than the orbicularis. It is a primary elevator of the lid and through the aponeurosis of its tendon attaches with the orbital septum to the anterior inferior aspect of the tarsus, the fibrous skeleton of the lid. The other primary elevator of the lid, Mueller's muscle, has sympathetic innervation and attaches to the retrotarsal margin. The frontalis and superior rectus muscles are secondary elevators of the lid and are indirectly attached to the tarsus; the frontalis is attached through the orbital septum, orbicularis and skin; the superior rectus is attached through fine fibrous bands to the upper cul-de-sac of the conjunctiva and to the levator and Mueller's muscles. The primary arteries of the upper lid lie in the pretarsal space. The marginal arcade runs along the edge of the lids and the peripheral arcade branches from the marginal arcade and follows the upper part of the tarsus.

Anatomical Variations Producing Ptosis

Congenital Abnormalities

1. It is possible but very rare for the levator to be absent.

2. The usual cause of ptosis is an abnormality in the structure or nerve supply of the levator muscle. Berke and Wadsworth* studied the levator tissue removed at the time of ptosis surgery. They found that in mild congenital ptosis (2 mm), striated muscle fibers were fewer than normal; in moderate ptosis (3 mm), the muscle fibers were seen in only 54 per cent of the cases; and in severe ptosis (4 mm or more), no striated muscle fibers were found. Accordingly, it could be postulated that the function of the muscle is inversely proportional to the replacement of its fibers by fibrous tissue. Isaksson† confirmed Berke and Wadsworth's findings and considered the changes a dystrophy. It has been debated whether these changes are a congenital abnormality, a dystrophy, or a sclerosis, but it makes no practical difference in the surgical handling of the condition.

In essence, if the resected portion of the aponeurosis and muscle taken at the time of surgery has fewer muscle fibers in relation to fibrous tissue, there is correspondingly less muscle to contract, and therefore the amplitude of contraction is reduced.

3. In some cases the nasal and lateral horns of the aponeurosis and Whitnall's ligament are so tight that they restrict the motion of the levator.

4. Faulty innervation of the levator muscle causes bizarre contractions called jaw-winking.

Acquired Abnormalities

1. The levator muscle may be separated from its attachment to the lid by trauma.

2. A spontaneous dehiscence can occur as seen in a senile ptosis.

3. The third nerve may be damaged or impaired by trauma, tumors, aneurysms or diabetes. The sympathetic nerve supply to Mueller's muscle may be damaged or impaired (Horner's syndrome).

4. The muscle may be involved in a dystrophy (progressive external ophthalmoplegia) or in generalized disease (scleroderma).

5. The muscle may be invaded by tumor or directly affected by some systemic disease, such as amyloidosis or myasthenia gravis.

TYPES OF PTOSIS

Our classification (Table 2–1) is not all-inclusive but is a working basis for the oculoplastic surgeon.

---

*Berke, R. N., and Wadsworth, J. A. C.: Histology of the levator muscle in congenital and acquired ptosis. Arch. Ophthal. 53:413, 1955.

†Isaksson, I.: Studies on congenital genuine blepharoptosis. *Acta Ophthalmologica* (Kbh), Suppl. 72, 1962.

TABLE 2–1. TYPES OF PTOSIS

Congenital
    Blepharophimosis—bilateral with epicanthal abnormalities
    Bilateral or unilateral without other abnormalities
    Bilateral or unilateral with superior rectus weakness
    Bilateral or unilateral with double elevator palsy
    Bilateral or unilateral with other ocular muscle anomalies
    Bilateral or unilateral with jaw-winking
    Horner's syndrome
    Ptosis with globe deformities

Acquired
    Mechanical
      Trauma
      Senile
      Tumor invasion
      Post-enucleation
      With dermachalasis
    Myogenic
      Progressive external ophthalmoplegia
      Oculopharyngeal syndrome
      Muscular dystrophy
      Late developing hereditary ptosis
    Neurogenic
      Post-inflammatory (diphtheria, encephalitis, meningitis, measles, etc.)
      Aneurysm
      Multiple sclerosis
      Myasthenia gravis
      Acquired Horner's syndrome
    Ptosis in association with systemic disease or of undertermined etiology

Ptosis to eliminate diplopia

Congenital Ptosis

Ptosis is considered congenital when it has existed from birth. It may be unilateral or bilateral and may be of varying severity. Over the years, the designation "congenital" has been repeatedly questioned. Whether correct or not, we use the word to mean that the ptosis is noted as soon as the infant has control of its ocular movements. Birth injury is often mentioned as a cause of the ptosis; if it is a cause, it is infrequent and has no effect on the choice of treatment.

Blepharophimosis. This condition is a hereditary dominant trait. The ptosis is always bilateral and has an associated narrowing of the lid fissures vertically and horizontally, epicanthus and variable degrees of ectropion of the lateral portions of the lower lids (Fig. 2–9). The horns of the aponeurosis are so tight that the lid edges may be stretched like bowstrings, making the upper lid difficult to evert. Because the thickened tissues of the lid make the eyes appear small, parents frequently think they are also abnormal. Operation on these children is difficult, and the results far from perfect.

Bilateral or Unilateral Ptosis Without Other Abnormalities. Congenital ptosis may be bilateral or unilateral and may vary from mild to severe. When it is bilateral, the child may just have a dreamy look or the lids may be so low that the head has to be tilted back for the visual axis to be cleared. These cases usually occur sporadically but may be familial. Unilateral congenital ptosis is encountered in all degrees and may be so severe as to produce a visual obstruction with the eyes in the straight-ahead position. With the eyes in the down position, however, the vision is not obstructed, and we have not found that deprivation amblyopia occurs. Since the infant's world depends on near vision, our observations seem logical.

When amblyopia has been found in association with unilateral ptosis, we have been able to demonstrate a defect in ocular motility, a refractive error, or some other abnormality to account for the poor vision (Fig. 2–10).

Bilateral or Unilateral Ptosis with Superior Rectus Muscle Weakness. Ptosis with an associated superior rectus malfunction is a muscular anomaly and not a neurological condition. Probably, the superior rectus muscle function is limited by the same kind of replacement of muscle fibers by fibrous tissue as occurs in the levator. Such ptosis is not infrequent and may be bilateral or unilateral, but unilateral is more common. Usually the eye will elevate to the primary position but no further. Forced duction tests easily elevate the eye further. The eyes move normally in the lower fields of gaze, and fusion is present. In these patients elevating the lid is quite satisfactory without any associated muscle surgery. On the other hand, some bilateral superior rectus anomalies are associated with a contraction of the inferior rectus muscles, in which case muscle surgery is necessary.

Bilateral or Unilateral Ptosis with Double Elevator Palsy. Double elevator palsy and ptosis may be unilateral (with homolateral ptosis and palsy) or bilateral. The patient is unable to elevate the eye past the primary position because of paresis of the superior rectus and inferior oblique muscles. The etiology is unknown, but preservation of Bell's phenomenon suggests a supranuclear lesion.

Bilateral or Unilateral Ptosis with Other Ocular Muscle Anomalies. When ptosis is associated with horizontal muscle anomalies, the muscle anomalies should be corrected first since a protective ptosis to avoid diplopia may persist in spite of any type of ptosis surgery. Therefore, an orthoptic workup should be done as soon as possible, and surgery or glasses prescribed as is indicated in any horizontal deviation. Following this, the ptosis can be corrected. Since the orbicularis muscle is many times more powerful than the levator, especially if the latter is abnormal, the lid will remain ptosed to avoid diplopia in spite of any operative procedure on the levator (Figs. 2–11 and 2–12). However, with congenital strabismus and ptosis, diplopia is usually not a problem and ptosis and horizontal muscle surgery can be done at the same time.

Jaw-winking (Marcus Gunn Phenomenon). Ten to 12 per cent of our patients with congenital ptosis exhibit the unilateral jaw-winking phenomenon; bilateral jaw-winking occurs but is rare. When the eyes are at rest in the primary position, there is a variable degree of ptosis of the involved lid (Fig. 2–13). The wink consists of a rapid elevation of the lid to a level often higher than the normal fellow lid (Fig. 2–14) and an almost equally rapid return to a less

Figures 2–9 to 2–16

Figure 2–9 Blepharophimosis and ptosis.

Figure 2–10 Ptosis and esotropia.

Figure 2–11 Ptosis remains after three attempts at repair. The protective etiology had gone unrecognized.

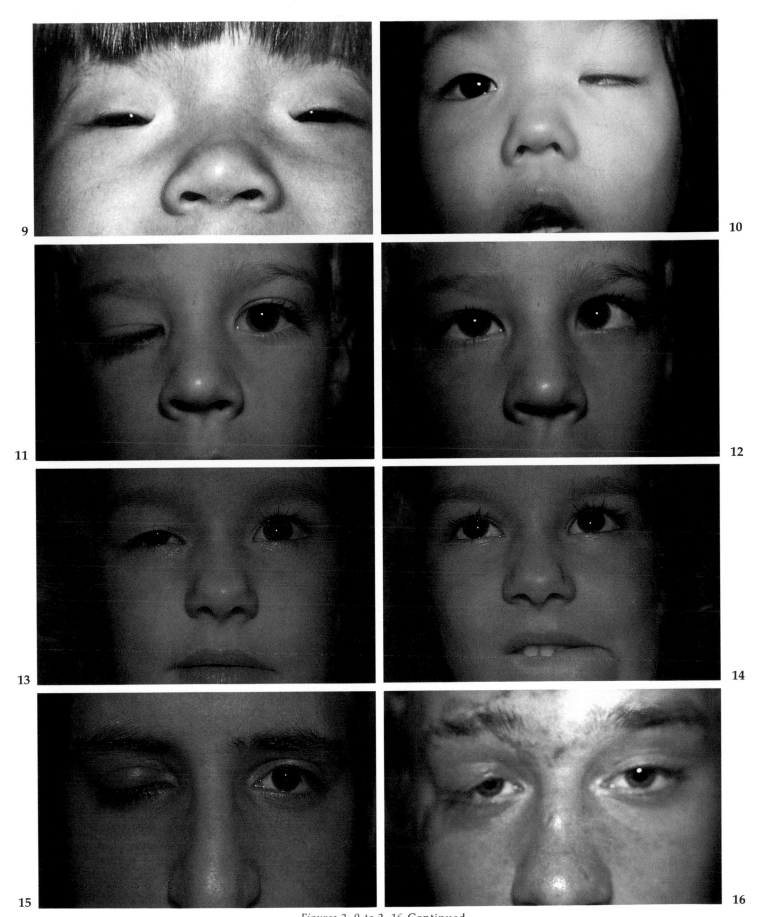

Figures 2–9 to 2–16 Continued

Figure 2–12   The child can raise the right lid voluntarily but has diplopia because of esotropia and 20/20 visual acuity in each eye.

Figures 2–13, 2–14   Jaw winker's ptosis temporally disappears with jaw motion.

Figure 2–15   Traumatic ptosis (complete).

Figure 2–16   Traumatic ptosis (partial).

29

elevated level. The lid may then remain for a time at the height of the normal lid or may droop to the original ptosed position. The rapidity of the motion produces a bizarre appearance that is disturbing to the patient and observers. The wink may be induced by sucking, swallowing, chewing, lateral motion of the jaw to either side or, in some cases, by extremes of gaze. In these patients, there is nothing wrong with the levator muscle, as the amplitude of motion and wink attest; why the lid droops is not apparent.

The patient, or the parents if the patient is too young to be consulted, and the ophthalmologist must choose whether the ptosis or the wink is the greater cosmetic blemish and which should be treated.

We feel the wink reflex will spontaneously decrease in a high percentage of cases. There have been relatively few adult jaw-winkers in our practice, in which 10 to 12 per cent of the children with ptosis have presented this feature. We have personally followed a number of patients in whom the wink decreased or disappeared. However, the original case of Marcus Gunn and one pictured in Figures 2–60 to 2–65 were young adults, and Berke and Beard* have both commented on seeing a number of adults with this condition.

Horner's Syndrome. Congenital Horner's syndrome is probably most commonly caused by trauma to the sympathetic fibers at the level of the brachial plexus at the time of birth. The levator muscle is presumably normal; therefore, the surgical approach is somewhat different from that used for "simple" congenital ptosis (see p. 43).

Ptosis with Globe Deformities. Ptosis may occur when there is enophthalmos or microphthalmus. There is loss of support and loss of a fulcrum around which the lid can rotate. Though the lid is ptotic secondary to an abnormality not connected with the lid (thus the term "pseudoptosis"), the appearance is the same as in "true" ptosis. The corrective measures can be directed at supplying the support not provided by the enophthalmic or microphthalmic globe; in addition, lid surgery may be necessary in selected instances.

Acquired Ptosis

MECHANICAL PTOSIS

That trauma can produce ptosis is easily understood. The levator muscle is detached, or its contraction is interfered with in reaching the lid. For example, a laceration occurring at the narrow portion of the muscle; or aponeurosis produces a complete ptosis (Fig. 2–15). Laceration occurring where the aponeurosis is wide may produce a nasal, middle, or lateral ptosis, depending on its extent (Fig. 2–16). Blunt trauma to the orbit frequently causes ptosis. Direct third cranial nerve damage (Fig. 2–17), hematoma, edema, and dehiscence of the levator muscle or tendon have all been incriminated. Blowout fracture with enophthalmus is a cause of secondary ptosis.

Senile ptosis has been puzzling for years; the etiology was not understood until Jones and Quickert† demonstrated dehiscences in

*Berke, R. N.: Personal communication; and Beard, C.: Personal communication.
†Jones, L. T., Quickert, M. H., and Wobig, J. L.: The cure of ptosis by aponeurotic repair. Arch. Ophthal. 93:629–34, August 1975.

the levator aponeurosis. In this, senile ptosis resembles traumatic ptosis, and repair of the aponeurosis is the treatment. Ptosis seen after intraocular operation seems to be in this category. In these patients, the horns are never tight, Whitnall's ligament does not restrict motion, and the muscle is not fibrotic. The ptosis differs from the congenital variety in that the lid shows the same degree of ptosis in primary, up, and down gaze.

Tumors of the lid (hemangiomas, neurofibromas, or dermolipomas) produce a mechanical restriction of the lid motion due to either the bulk of the tumor or invasion of the lid tissues and levator muscle (Fig 2–18). Treatment is discussed in Chapter 9; the surgeon must exercise great care and restraint so that removal of the tumor does not harm the patient more than would the tumor if left alone.

Ptosis following the enucleation of an eye may result from damage to the levator muscle or to its nerve or may be due to a poorly fitting prosthesis that does not present a fulcrum for the levator muscle to act against. If the latter, a new prosthesis should be tried.

A ptosis associated with a small or phthisical eye is best treated with a cosmetic contact lens and, if necessary, minimal lid surgery.

Ptosis associated with dermochalasis requires a blepharoplasty in addition to the elevation of the lid.

Myogenic Ptosis

Progressive external ophthalmoplegia produces complete immobility of the globes. The levator is weakened, producing a ptosis, but the orbicularis is usually not involved until very late in the disease so voluntary closing of the eyes is not hampered.

Late hereditary ptosis is familial, begins between the ages of forty and fifty years, and may be a part of the oculopharyngeal syndrome.

Neurogenic Ptosis

Myasthenia gravis patients can be helped by ptosis surgery that complements their general medical therapy. Most cases of neurogenic ptosis, however, are of more interest to the neurophthalmologist as a diagnostic sign than to the oculoplastic surgeon.

Ptosis from Unknown Etiology

The etiology of some forms of acquired ptosis is often obscure. That acute illnesses, such as measles, influenza, encephalitis, and meningitis, can cause ptosis is suspected but difficult to prove. The ptosis of adolescence fits into this unexplained category.

Ptosis to Eliminate Diplopia

Protective ptosis occurs when a patient voluntarily closes the lid to relieve an annoying diplopia. No surgical procedure on the lid will correct the ptosis until the diplopia is cured. (See Figs. 2–11 and 2–12.)

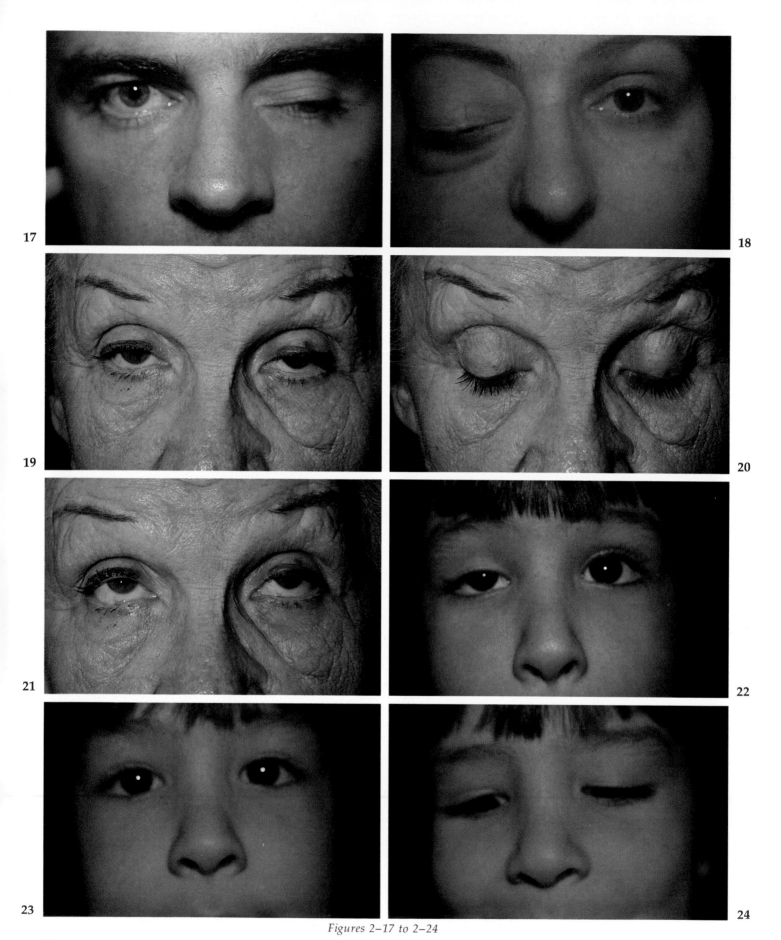

Figures 2–17 to 2–24

Figure 2–17 Traumatic third nerve palsy.
Figure 2–18 Hemangioma of right orbit.
Figures 2–19, 2–20, 2–21 Bilateral senile ptosis.

Figure 2–22 Preoperative congenital ptosis.
Figure 2–23 Postoperative congenital ptosis.
Figure 2–24 Lid lag on operated eye in down gaze.

PREOPERATIVE CONSIDERATIONS

History

A good history is important in the management of ptosis, as in any surgery. Although the surgical approach may not be altered by the history, it is still necessary to rule out neurological or systemic disorders that may require additional attention.

Time of onset, abruptness of presentation, any associated symptoms, and whether the ptosis is intermittent or variable should be determined. Myasthenia gravis has to be considered, even in children, and if it is suspected, a Tensilon test should be done. Particularly in adults, history of diplopia, headache, or diabetes is significant. Trauma, ocular irritation, infection, or previous ophthalmic surgery may be contributing factors. Family history of ocular disease is pertinent.

Ptosis surgery in any patient with a history of dry eyes should be approached with extreme caution.

It is important to record any such symptoms that are present preoperatively, for if they persist the patient may attribute them to the surgery. During the history taking and physical examination, an evaluation of the mental and emotional status of the patient should be done, for this may have a bearing on the advisability of surgery.

In considering surgery, it is important to know if the patient has had general or local anesthesia and how it was tolerated. Have there been any adverse reactions, such as malignant hyperthermia, to anesthesia in parents or other family members?

It is important to record visual or asthenopic components associated with even a slight degree of ptosis, although the reason for correcting a ptosis in most instances is a cosmetic one. In the acquired or secondary ptoses — senile, traumatic, and those associated with general disease or tumors — vision is often affected; even patients with a very slight ptosis may have a visual problem.

Examination

A photograph in the primary position and in up and downward gaze is helpful. In a senile ptosis, the lid remains in the same ptotic position relative to the globe in all levels of gaze (Figs. 2–19 to 2–21). In a congenital ptosis, there is often restriction of motion of the lid on downward gaze producing a relative lid lag in both upward and downward gaze. A photograph of the preoperative lid lag is good to have because shortening the levator tendon will make the lag more apparent on downward gaze (Figs. 2-22 to 2-24). If the surgeon has not pointed out the lid lag to the parents as a preoperative finding, they will certainly point it out to him postoperatively.

Examination should include tests of vision and refraction, measurement of ocular tension, fundus examination, orthoptic work-up, an estimation of the amount of ptosis and levator function, a

Actual
Berke and V
lines, for un
timated as
more) (Fig.
(8 mm or n
be absent.
the globe.
and ability
levator. It i
tion of the
bined with
with fair to
This ki
tient, and u
tion can be
have an aw
correction.
genital pto
to learn to
tremely po
child is a g

*Berke, R.
acquired ptosis
†Beard, C.

In addition to levator function, degree of ptosis, and contour of the lids, the tightness of the horns and Whitnall's check ligament must be determined at the time of surgery.

Conditions that May Contraindicate Ptosis Surgery

The dry eye or keratitis sicca as indicated by a low Schirmer test (less than 4 to 5 mm in 5 minutes) may have produced a protective or irritative ptosis. Although this condition is much more frequent in adults, it occasionally occurs in children. Occlusion of the puncta as described under lacrimal surgery (Chapter 6) may conserve the available tears to give a comfortable eye. This may relieve the ptosis completely if it has been a reaction to irritation of the dry eye or may make the patient a candidate for surgical elevation of the lid at least above the visual axis.

Infrequent blinking is often associated with loss of or decrease in corneal sensitivity, and a study of the tear film pattern should be carefully done before ptosis surgery is advised. Decreased or lost corneal sensitivity should make the surgeon wary. In these cases if elevation of the lid is necessary for visual purposes, it should only be high enough to clear the visual axis.

Certainly if the eye is fixed by some infiltrative process, such as scleroderma, or by a neuropathy or myopathy that keeps the globe from moving, the elevation of a ptosed lid by surgery must be done with caution. However, if the orbicularis is still working and there is a good blink reflex and normal corneal sensitivity, it is feasible to elevate the lid to clear the visual axis.

Sometimes Bell's phenomenon has been confused with the erratic motion of the eyes during sleep. Bell's phenomenon is a protective mechanism in which the eyes roll upward with forceful defensive closure of the lids. When Bell's phenomenon is absent, it is, of course, possible that foreign bodies could damage the cornea and that elevating the lids might increase this danger. We have not found this to be a problem and do not consider the absence of a Bell's phenomenon to be a contraindication to surgery. More important is the fact that in progressive external ophthalmoplegia the eyes do not roll up under the lids in sleep nor do they exhibit the normal erratic motion during sleep; thus corneal drying occurs unless ointment is applied to the cornea and the lids are closed at night with plastic tape. These patients have true lagophthalmos (not to be confused — as many ophthalmologists have done — with lid lag), which Webster's International Dictionary, Unabridged Second Edition, gives as derived from "*lagōs* hare + *ophthalmos* eye; from the notion that a hare sleeps with his eyes open" and defines as "a morbid condition in which the eye does not completely close, giving a peculiar staring appearance."

If, from history or examination, myasthenia gravis is suspected, a Tensilon test should be performed. If the test is positive, therapy is planned cooperatively by the internist and the oculoplastic surgeon.

Summary

In ptosis surgery, as in any surgery, history is important. Strabismus, trauma, previous surgery, and systemic or neurological disorders are significant. Knowledge of a patient's past response to anesthesia is basic.

A history of visual disturbance, asthenopia, dry eyes, or ocular irritation may markedly affect management, not to mention the patient's expectations and understanding of the problem.

Examination begins with a complete routine ophthalmic examination. Measurement of intraocular pressure and adequate fundus examination in children can be deferred to the time of surgery, but should not be forgotten. If amblyopia is present, look for strabismus or anisometropia, as amblyopia is extremely rare (if it ever occurs) on the basis of "simple" ptosis alone. The ptosis is evaluated by determining the level of the lid (which often can only be estimated) and levator function as indicated by lid fold, lid excursion on up and downward gaze while the brow is immobilized, and by the return on upgaze of an everted lid to its usual position. Gum chewing may be helpful in detecting jaw-winking. Treatment of dry eyes or those with abnormal tear film should be approached cautiously.

The possibility of infiltrative processes, neuropathies, and myopathies should not be forgotten. Third nerve palsy and myasthenia gravis should be kept in mind during evaluation of a ptosis patient. The absence of Bell's phenomenon is not a contraindication to surgery.

THE CHOICE OF OPERATION

The amplitude of contraction of the levator muscle in a normal lid is about 15 mm. In a congenital ptosis this may be reduced. Eight mm or more is considered good; 5 to 7 mm, fair; and less than 4 mm, poor (Table 2–2).

In a congenital ptosis if there is no levator muscle contraction, a frontalis sling should be done. If there is demonstrable levator contraction, a levator aponeurosis shortening procedure should be done. The obvious question is how much shortening of the aponeurosis is necessary to correct each millimeter of ptosis? We have used as a working guide a 6 to 1 ratio — resecting approximately 6 mm of aponeurosis to obtain 1 mm of lid elevation. Thus, if we have a mild congenital

TABLE 2–2. CHOICE OF OPERATION

Amount of Ptosis	Levator Contraction Amplitude	Levator Resection
Normal (no ptosis)	Excellent, 15 mm	– –
Mild, 1 to 2 mm	Good, 8 mm or more	10 to 12 mm
Moderate, 3 mm	Fair, 5 to 7 mm	18 mm
Severe, 4 mm	Poor, less than 4 mm	24 mm
Severe, 4 mm or more	None, 0	Frontalis sling

ptosis (1 to 2 mm), the resection of the aponeurosis would be 6 to 12 mm; if a moderate ptosis of 3 mm, the resection would be 18 mm; and for a severe 4 mm ptosis, 24 mm of resection. However, the relationship is not entirely linear, and for mild degrees of ptosis (1 to 2 mm), a 10 to 12 mm resection gives the best result.

The Fasanella-Servat operation resects in block conjunctiva, tarsus and levator aponeurosis. The amount of tarsus that can safely be resected limits this operation to the correction of a mild ptosis of 1 to 2 mm only. Our procedure consists of a resection above the retrotarsal margin so that a larger ptosis can be treated and the tarsus is not compromised.

Resecting the relatively inelastic aponeurosis can elevate the lid but does not increase the amplitude of the muscle contraction. Thus if you have a 3 mm ptosis with 5 to 7 mm of amplitude of contraction, shortening the aponeurosis will elevate the range of motion of the lid and correct the ptosis in the primary straight-ahead position — but the amplitude of motion will still be 5 to 7 mm, so that on downward gaze the lid follow will be less than preoperatively.

In some patients the horns and Whitnall's ligament will be found at the time of operation to be restricting the motion of the levator muscle. Cutting these can free the muscle and increase its amplitude of contraction.

Our operative plan has been to shorten the levator aponeurosis and Mueller's muscle by doing a small "block resection" of 6 to 12 mm for a mild ptosis, a large "block resection" of 18 mm for moderate ptosis, and a maximum levator resection of 24 mm with cutting of the horns and Whitnall's ligament for a severe ptosis. This has seemed to be a fairly workable yardstick for our ptosis surgery. The amount of resection is decided preoperatively; the decision whether to cut the horns and Whitnall's ligament is made at the time of operation.

From the history and examination, the surgeon can choose which operation will be the most effective and decide when it should be done. The history will have indicated whether the ptosis is congenital or acquired, and the examination will have demonstrated how well the levator is functioning. The amplitude of function of the levator is important in predicting the cosmetic success of the operation. Obviously, good levator function gives a better result.

There are two acceptable methods for elevating the lid and creating a good lid fold. If there is no levator action, the lid is suspended from the frontalis muscle using autogenous or preserved fascia lata placed as a double rhomboid sling from the frontalis to the lid. If there is some levator action, the lid is elevated by shortening the levator tendon.

Congenital Ptosis

BLEPHAROPHIMOSIS

Bilateral blepharophimosis and bilateral severe ptosis are corrected with bilateral frontalis slings. An infant with bilateral severe ptosis should be operated upon as soon as he is considered a good anesthesia risk. The best time, we feel, is between 9 months and 1 year, before the ptosis (producing the head-back position) jeopardizes learning to walk (Fig. 2–26). With a large ptosis and no levator muscle function, levator resection is inadequate for normal lid position and lid function. Therefore, the procedure of choice is bilateral frontalis slings. Normal lid position is easily obtained, and some dynamic function is provided by the frontalis muscle.

Children with blepharophimosis have bilateral ptosis, narrowed lid fissures, and distorted epicanthal areas. The horns are extremely tight and occasionally the tissues of the lid are thickened. Operation on these children is difficult. Levator shortening procedures are much less satisfactory than a frontalis sling; therefore, a sling is routinely done at about one year of age. The epicanthal abnormalities are usually left alone at this time and correction postponed until shortly before puberty when the child will have developed more bridge to the nose, which tends to decrease the deformity.

Frontalis Sling. In infants, Crawford's preserved human fascia (obtainable from The Department of Ophthalmology, University of Toronto) is used, as it is difficult to get autogenous fascia long enough for two lids from one leg. Autogenous fascia can be used in older children. If the preserved fascia fails, it usually does so within the first three months because of the absorption of the fascia. A repeat of the procedure using preserved fascia does not seem to be jeopardized by the first failure, but in most instances we will delay a second operation until autogenous fascia can be taken.

We agree with Beard that a frontalis sling should be a bilateral procedure to give the best static and dynamic symmetry of the lids. The exceptions to this are in patients with a complete ptosis of an enucleated eye and in patients with a severe ptosis from trauma, nerve or muscle damage, or tumor invasion who wish some cosmetic improvement but realize that perfection is impossible. If operations are to be done on both upper lids, they should be done at the same time, as it is easier that way to judge the equality of the two procedures. In some instances it may be desirable to increase the tension of the sling in the more ptotic lid in an attempt to equalize the results.

The utilization of the superior rectus muscle has no advantage over the frontalis sling or a levator shortening procedure and has the disadvantage of producing a vertical muscle imbalance, which can cause an annoying diplopia and, in some instances, cause an exposure keratitis that is difficult to overcome. For these reasons, we feel its use is never indicated.

BILATERAL OR UNILATERAL PTOSIS
WITHOUT OTHER ABNORMALITIES

Bilateral or unilateral ptosis with some levator function is treated with one of several levator shortening procedures depending on the severity of the ptosis.

Mild (1 to 2 mm) Congenital Ptosis (Fig. 2–27) — Small Block Resection (Iliff). Conjunctiva, Mueller's muscle, and levator aponeurosis are resected in block. The tarsus is not disturbed so that lid curve is not distorted and peaking of the lid margin is less likely to occur. The exception is a partial tarsectomy when the tarsus is found to be wider

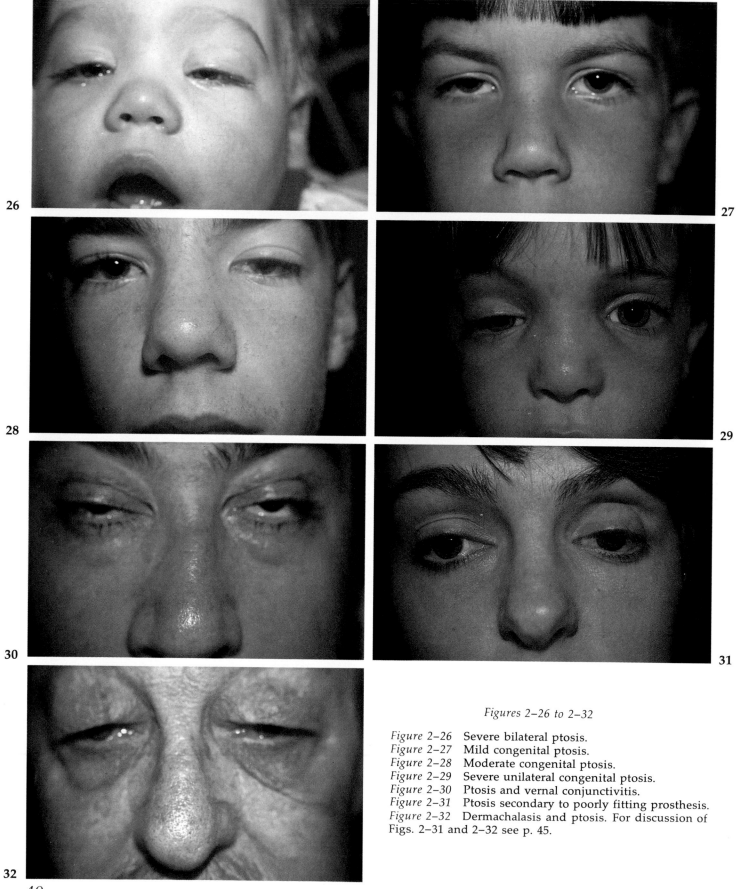

Figures 2–26 to 2–32

Figure 2–26   Severe bilateral ptosis.
Figure 2–27   Mild congenital ptosis.
Figure 2–28   Moderate congenital ptosis.
Figure 2–29   Severe unilateral congenital ptosis.
Figure 2–30   Ptosis and vernal conjunctivitis.
Figure 2–31   Ptosis secondary to poorly fitting prosthesis.
Figure 2–32   Dermachalasis and ptosis. For discussion of
Figs. 2–31 and 2–32 see p. 45.

than normal laterally, giving a droop to this portion of the lid. In such cases, we have found that a lateral resection of 2 to 3 mm of tarsus is helpful in correcting the defect.

Ten to 12 mm of conjunctiva, Mueller's muscle and levator aponeurosis can be removed, giving predictable results. The proximal edge of the levator aponeurosis is reattached to its original insertion. Mueller's muscle and conjunctiva are attached to their original insertions. The operation is an anatomical and physiological one. Because of the reattachment of the levator to its original insertion we have not encountered postoperative downward turning of the cilia, or the postoperative corneal irritation that occurs because of suture placement with some of the Fasanella-Servat type operations.

Moderate (3 mm) Congenital Ptosis (Fig. 2–28) — Large Block Resection (Iliff). Eighteen mm of levator aponeurosis can be resected by increasing the tension on the traction sutures placed in the aponeurosis before the holding sutures are inserted. A greater piece of aponeurosis can then be excised.

Severe (4 mm) Unilateral Ptosis (Fig. 2–29) — Maximum Levator Resection Through the Conjunctiva (Iliff). Conjunctiva is spared; the horns and Whitnall's ligament are cut. Twenty-four mm of aponeurosis and muscle can be excised, and the proximal edge of the muscle resutured to its original insertion on the anterior lower one third of the tarsus.

In senile ptosis, the lid is equally ptotic with respect to the globe in up and downward gaze; in congenital ptosis, however, there is frequently restriction of the lid and consequent lid lag in downward gaze. It must be understood that resection of the inelastic levator muscle will further restrict the lid follow on downward gaze. Shortening the tendon of a fibrotic levator muscle in congenital ptosis elevates the primary lid position but does not change the amplitude of the excursion. On the other hand, cutting Whitnall's ligament and tight horns, which are restricting the motion of the muscle, may well increase the muscle action.

Maximum Levator Resection — Anterior Skin Route (Berke). We have used the anterior or skin approach when it facilitates the removal of a lid tumor or when the conjunctiva has been involved in some pathology (Fig. 2–30). It is also used if a failure has occurred with a conjunctival approach, in which case it is much easier to go above the scarring at the retrotarsal margin and resect the aponeurosis at a higher level through the skin approach.

BILATERAL OR UNILATERAL PTOSIS WITH SUPERIOR RECTUS MUSCLE WEAKNESS

Congenital bilateral ptosis with associated superior rectus palsy is an uncommon condition compared to unilateral ptosis with associated superior rectus involvement.

If the eyes can be elevated to a straight-ahead gaze and limitation is above the horizontal only, no muscle surgery is necessary at the time of the lid surgery. The operation is a levator shortening procedure, governed by the amount of levator action.

If the eyes are fixed in the downward gaze, elevating the lids gives a bizarre, unreal appearance and may cause a corneal breakdown. If the

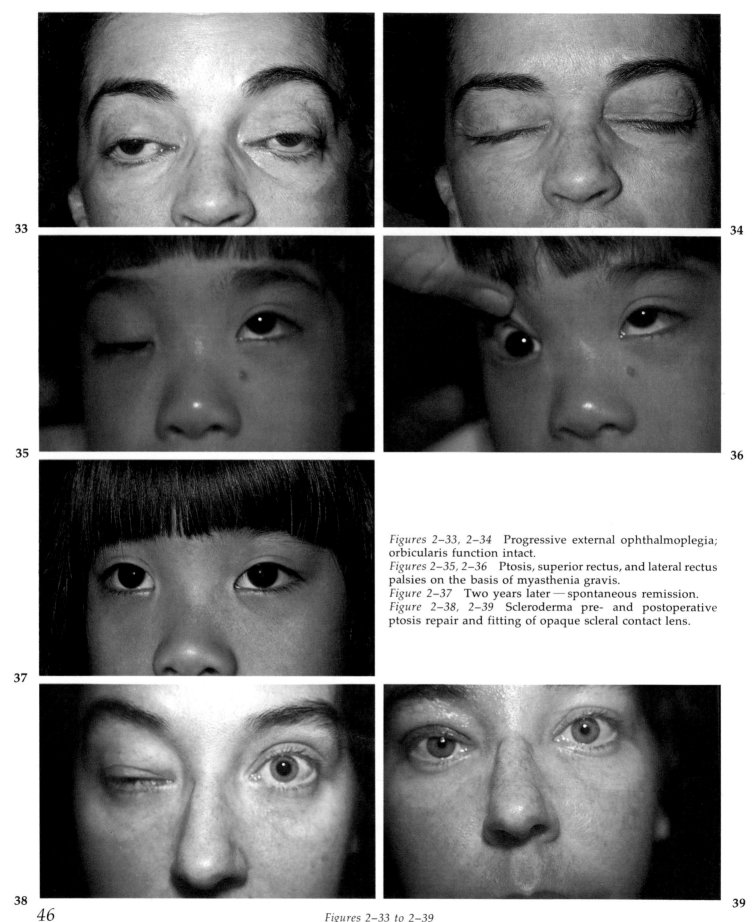

Figures 2–33, 2–34 Progressive external ophthalmoplegia; orbicularis function intact.

Figures 2–35, 2–36 Ptosis, superior rectus, and lateral rectus palsies on the basis of myasthenia gravis.

Figure 2–37 Two years later — spontaneous remission.

Figure 2–38, 2–39 Scleroderma pre- and postoperative ptosis repair and fitting of opaque scleral contact lens.

Figures 2–33 to 2–39

PTOSIS ASSOCIATED WITH SYSTEMIC
DISEASE OR WITH AN UNDETERMINED
ETIOLOGY

Scleroderma. The levator is usually involved along with ocular muscles, and the elevation of the lid may produce an annoying diplopia (Figs. 2–38, 2–39). Therefore, surgery will be unsuccessful no matter what method is used unless the vision of one eye is blanked out with a cosmetic scleral contact lens. Depending on the amount of ptosis, some kind of block or levator resection is indicated.

Ptosis in the Young Adult. The ptosis of adolescence or young adult life is of unknown etiology. Surgery is based on the measured amount of ptosis but should be relatively conservative. Rarely is more than a large block resection needed.

Keratitis Sicca. If the patient has symptoms of dry eyes, surgery for ptosis should, of course, be approached with extreme caution. If an operation is necessary to clear the visual axis, a small block resection may be done if there is levator function or a minimal frontalis sling using Supramid if there is no levator function. In either case, the surgeon should strive to raise the lids just above the visual axis.

SUMMARY

In congenital ptosis, the amount of levator to be resected can be determined through guidelines that take into account the preoperative measurements and the effect of the horns and Whitnall's ligament as evaluated at surgery.

A severe bilateral ptosis in which there is no levator action requires a frontalis sling, which should be done as soon as the child is a good risk for anesthesia.

In patients who have some levator function, surgery is postponed to the age of 3 to 4. At this point, the patient often can cooperate for more extensive evaluation.

Strabismus can be repaired at the same time as the ptosis provided the two procedures do not have overlapping incisions. Therefore, a frontalis sling can be done with any strabismus surgery. If horizontal muscle surgery is done through inferior forniceal incisions, the procedure can be combined with any of the ptosis repairs. However, in general it is preferable to repair any horizontal strabismus prior to ptosis surgery.

Senile ptosis can usually be treated by a small block resection. The other kinds of acquired ptosis require individual evaluation and an approach tailored to each situation.

After enucleation or in a patient with a shrunken or enophthalmic eye, ptosis is caused by a loss of a fulcrum for the lid. A proper shell or prosthesis often solves the problem. Ptosis caused by or in conjunction with blepharochalasis requires correction of both conditions. Patients with progressive external ophthalmoplegia or dry eyes should be carefully evaluated and their lids raised only enough to clear the visual axis. If a sling is required, it is advisable to use a material that can be removed, such as Supramid, rather than fascia lata.

OPERATIVE TECHNIQUE

Frontalis Sling

The upper lid is suspended from the frontalis muscle at the level of the orbital rim where the muscle has its greatest amplitude of contraction (Fig. 2–40). This fastens the lid margin to the brow, elevating and lowering it as the brow moves up and down. Tension on the sling produces a lid crease, and the upper edge of the tarsus is rolled backward over the globe (Figs. 2–41 and 2–42). Since the frontalis muscle is a secondary elevator of the lid and is normally used by the patient in trying to raise the ptotic lid, the surgery merely aids a natural movement by giving a firmer connection between the lid and brow with an inelastic sling material. The cosmetic result is good (Fig. 2–43) with the exception that the lid-follow of the globe on down gaze is not complete (Fig. 2–44). Because of this limitation, a unilateral frontalis sling is cosmetically less satisfactory.

Beard* some years ago made the suggestion that both upper lids — the normal and the ptotic — should have a sling to create dynamic as well as static symmetry. This advanced approach was not accepted for a time but is now used almost universally and gives an excellent result. The bilateral sling is cosmetically pleasing and allows coordinated movements of the lids as they follow the

*Beard, C.: *Ptosis,* 2nd Ed., St. Louis, C. V. Mosby Co., 1976.

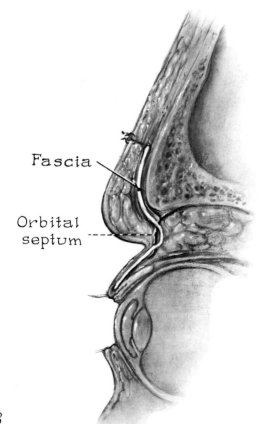

Fascia

Orbital septum

Figure 2–40

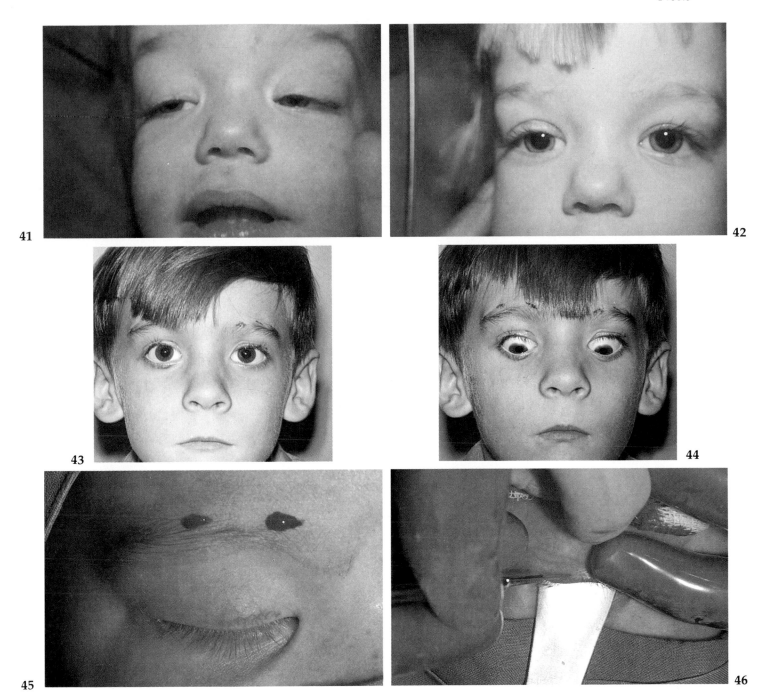

Figures 2–41 to 2–46

Figures 2–41 and 2–42 Preoperative and postoperative frontalis sling.
Figures 2–43 and 2–44 Postoperative frontalis sling; lid lag is present.
Figures 2–45 and 2–46 Brow and lid margin incisions. See p. 52 for discussion of frontalis sling procedure.

globe in the up and down positions even though there is limitation on down gaze.

The operation using the frontalis muscle is not new, but when reintroduced by Guyton and Friedenwald,* it attained popularity and because of its simplicity was used as an operation for all ptosis problems by many who had not been doing ptosis surgery. Braided, twisted, or woven silk, tantalum, silver wire, steel, catgut, collagen, and more recently Silastic and Supramid have all been used. Glowing reports of the immediate success of these fill the literature; however, with the exception of Supramid, which may not have been in use long enough to be evaluated, all have a high failure rate. Early and late infections are encountered and the sling material either stretches, cuts through the supporting tissues, is absorbed, or acts as a foreign body and has to be removed.

Supramid,** according to Byron Smith,† does not have as high a failure rate as Silastic; it remains apart from the surrounding tissue and, unlike fascia, can be removed if necessary. Its use is recommended if a trial suspension is necessary to determine whether the cornea will tolerate correction of the ptosis. This might be the case in ptosis of neurogenic origin, in ptosis associated with systemic disease such as scleroderma, or following trauma in which a waiting period is desired to see if levator function returns.

Surgeons who do a lot of ptosis surgery agree that autogenous fascia lata is the most reliable material for the sling. It gives perfect support, is ultimately integrated into its new environment, and does not produce late complications. The rejection rate is low and infections are rare.

There are some disadvantages to autogenous fascia lata. A separate operative procedure is necessary to obtain the fascia, prolonging the anesthetization time. In young children, it is difficult to get enough fascia from one leg to do both upper lids. A small scar results in the outer lower portion of the thigh. Placement and tying are slightly more difficult with fascia than with Supramid.

Crawford has helped to avoid the disadvantages of fascia lata by (1) developing a fascia stripper (Storz No. N-4298) (Fig. 2–47) for the

*Friedenwald, J. S., and Guyton, J. S.: A simplified ptosis operation: utilization of the frontalis by means of a single rhomboid-shaped suture. Am. J. Ophthal. 31:411, April 1948.
**Supramid is available on a long needle from S. Jackson, Inc. (2GS-2-40).
†Personal communication.

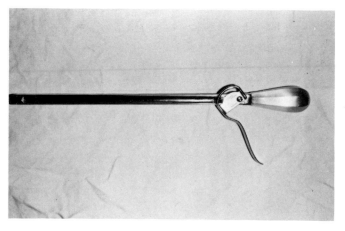

Figure 2–47

surgeon to use in removing autogenous fascia and (2) by preparing a preserved human fascia lata — which we have used since 1969, with excellent results. When an occasional failure does occur with preserved fascia, it is in the first few months and seems to be based on absorption of the material. When a failure has occurred, we have repeated the procedure with autogenous fascia and have had good results.

The frontalis sling operation presented here reduces the difficulty of the procedure and, in our opinion, makes the fascia lata, preserved or autogenous, the material of choice.

OPERATION TO OBTAIN AUTOGENOUS FASCIA LATA

Following the induction of general anesthesia, the fascia lata of the leg is put on stretch by slightly bending the knee and turning it inward and turning the heel outward. A pillow is placed beneath the hip and between the legs, and a piece of adhesive tape is placed across the lower leg to hold the knee in position. The skin of the lateral surface of the thigh is prepared with povidone-iodine (Betadine) from the knee to the upper portion of the thigh.

A horizontal incision, 5 cm long, is made over the fascia, approximately 2.5 to 5.0 cm above the lateral condyle, depending on the age and size of the patient. (If the incision is too close to the condyle, the fibers of fascia have a random pattern.) The incision is carried through skin, subcutaneous tissue, and fat to the fascia, which can be seen as a white, glistening, heavy sheet of tissue with fibers running parallel to the axis of the leg. Two skin rakes are used to give exposure. The fascia is picked up with Adson skin forceps, and a 1 cm full depth incision perpendicular to the fibers is made with scissors. One cut parallel to the fibers is made at each end of the transverse incision; each cut is extended proximally for approximately 2 cm. A 4–0 black silk suture is fastened to the end of the fascia to mobilize the lower end and to facilitate threading it into the Crawford stripper.

The sharp lateral cutting edges of the stripper split the fascia along the parallel fibers with relative ease. Tension is put on the skin below the end of the stripper as it is passed along the tendon with a push-retract advancement. At the 25 cm level, the lever is closed to cut the fascia, and the stripper and fascia are withdrawn. The subcutaneous tissue of this incision is closed with 4–0 chromic catgut, and the skin is closed with a vertical mattress suture of 4–0 silk. An elastic bandage (Ace) is applied to the thigh, and for 2 days the patient's activities are restricted to avoid a late hemorrhage. Usually, little postoperative reaction or pain is experienced. The skin sutures are removed after 8 days.

The excised fascia strip is pinned on a board to hold it on stretch. Clinging fat and subcutaneous tissue are removed. The strip of fascia, which now is approximately 8 mm wide, is split for its full length, great care being taken to separate the fibers with straight scissors, cutting across as few as possible. This will give two excellent strips approximately 3 to 4 mm wide and 25 cm long, which will be enough to do both lids.

As a rule, general anesthesia is used for children and local anesthesia for adults — except if fascia is to be taken from the leg, when general anesthesia is used for both adults and children. Local anesthesia consists of injection of 2 to 4 cc of 1 per cent lidocaine beneath the skin across the brow, and 1 to 2 cc across the lid at the level of the lid fold.

OPERATION: FRONTALIS SLING

Three deep stab incisions, 2.5 mm long, are made with a No. 15 Bard-Parker knife at the upper edge of the cilia of the brow. The lateral incision is made first because the brow is extremely vascular, and if either the nasal or the middle incision is made first, the blood will flow temporally and obscure the operative field. The lateral incision is made at the upper cilia edge 0.5 cm above the bony orbital rim and directly above the lateral canthus. The middle incision is made at the same level above the center of the lid and the nasal incision above the inner canthus (Fig. 2–45, p. 49). Pressure is exerted over the three incisions by the assistant to produce hemostasis while the lid incisions are made.

A lid plate (Storz No. E-2504) is covered with ointment and placed under the lid. Three horizontal stab incisions 2 mm long are made 1 mm above the cilia line, through the skin and the pretarsal muscle, down to the tarsus (Fig. 2–46, p. 49). The temporal incision is placed 6 mm from the lateral canthus, the middle incision is in the center of the lid, and the nasal incision is 6 mm from the medial canthus. Sharp-pointed scissors (iris spring action) are used to undermine the skin between these incisions to facilitate the passage of the fascia. A small hemostat is passed to the base of each brow incision and is spread to create a wide base for the seating of fascia (Fig. 2–49).

An empty Wright needle (Storz No. E-954) is inserted into the middle brow incision to the depth of the periosteum. It is passed down at this depth across the orbital rim behind the orbital septum and brought out superficially into the lid anterior to the tarsal plate, to emerge through the middle lid incision (Fig. 2–50). The fascia is threaded through the needle until the center of the strip is reached; the Wright needle is then withdrawn, pulling the doubled fascia through the middle lid incision and out the middle brow incision. To prevent cilia from being pulled into the tract with the fascia, which would increase the possibility of infection, a cotton swab applicator is used to hold them away from the fascia as it is being pulled through the tunnel (Fig. 2–51). The doubled fascia is cut at the needle, making the two equal-length strips that will be used to produce the two supporting rhomboids.

The empty Wright needle is inserted in the temporal lid incision and is passed beneath the skin to the middle lid incision. The

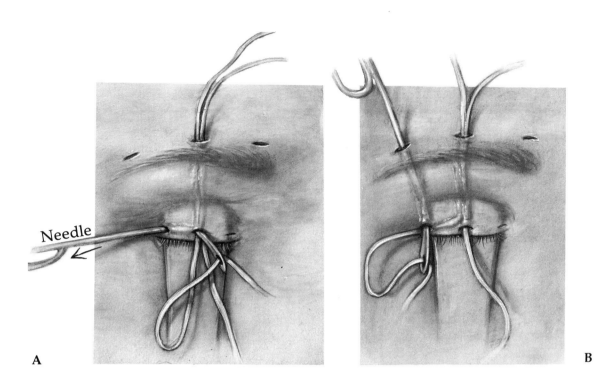

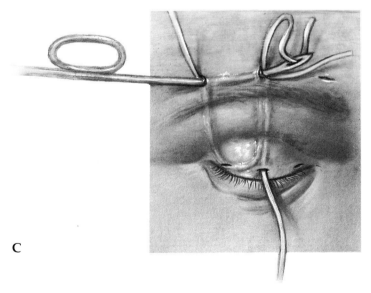

Figure 2–48

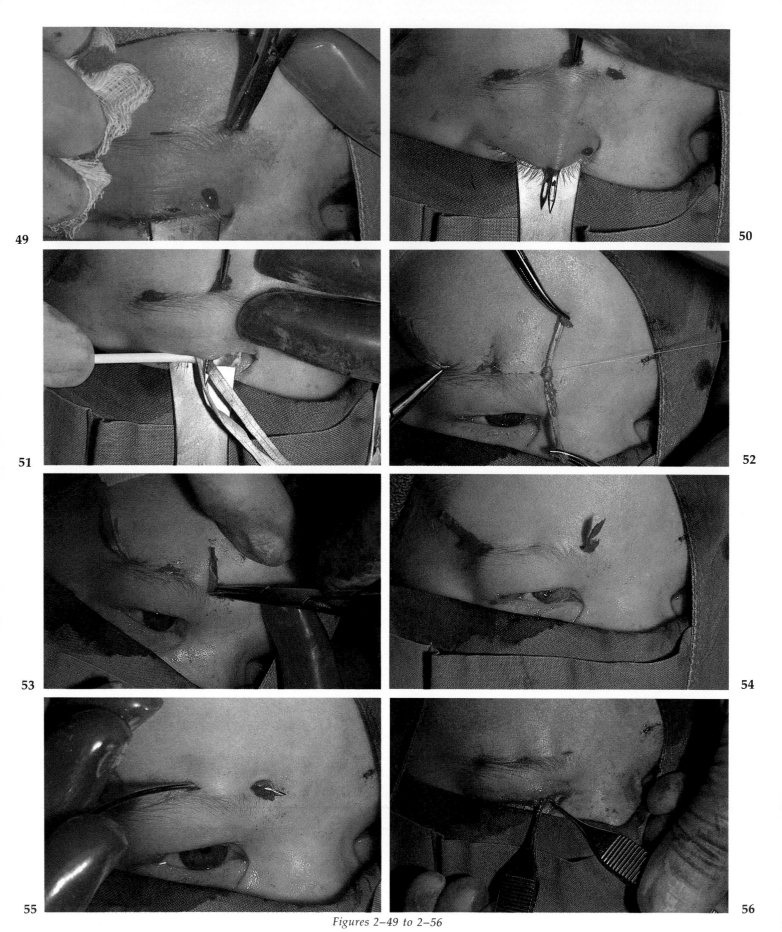

49 **50** **51** **52** **53** **54** **55** **56**

Figures 2–49 to 2–56

54   *Figure 2–49*   Hemostat is used to make pocket for fascial knot.

Figures 2–50 and 2–51   Wright needle inserted and fascial strip threaded.

Figure 2–52   A single tie is secured with suture.

Figure 2–53   Fascial tie is buried.

Figures 2–54 and 2–55   Fascial ends are buried.

Figure 2–56   Lid contour is adjusted.

end of one fascial strand is threaded through the needle for about 5 mm and is drawn out through the temporal lid incision (Fig. 2–48A). The needle is then directed from the temporal brow incision downward behind the orbital septum and out through the temporal lid incision. The fascia is threaded into the eye of the needle and drawn out in a similar manner through the temporal brow incision (Fig. 2–48B). Again, the needle is passed from the same temporal brow incision to the middle brow incision and the opposite end of the same fascial strand is threaded into the eye of the needle and pulled out through the temporal brow incision (Fig. 2–48C). This produces the temporal rhomboid, and the tension on the two ends will elevate the lateral half of the lid. The same steps are carried out in the same order to complete the medial rhomboid, using the second strip of fascia.

By using the two strands of fascia in this fashion, the middle as well as the temporal and nasal portions of the lid can be controlled to produce a good lid curve, which is normally slightly higher in the nasal one third than in the temporal (Fig. 2–57A).

By having the fascia fastened to the subcutaneous tissue and pretarsal muscle rather than to the tarsus, the lashes get an uplift. Passing the sling back through the orbital septum keeps the tarsus from being pulled away from the globe when the frontalis contracts; it is rolled naturally upward and backward over the globe in its normal travel.

Both strands of fascia are pulled sufficiently tight to produce a good lid fold and to elevate the lid so it crosses the upper limbus with the eye in the primary position.

The ends of the fascia projecting from the nasal brow incision are grasped with small curved hemostats and a single tie is placed, pulling the fascia tight enough to produce an immediate overcorrection, which is necessary as relaxation occurs when the knot is pushed into the incision. Tension is held on the hemostats while a 5–0 absorbable suture is used to secure the single fascial tie by several through-and-through bites and a firm knot (Fig. 2–52). The fascia is extremely slippery and a single tie will not hold unless fastened in this manner; a square knot is too bulky. The ends of the fascia are left long, projecting from the wound. The tie is grasped with a hemostat and is pushed into the base of the incision so that it will be well buried in the pocket that was made at the time of the original brow incision (Fig. 2–53). The fascia projecting from the temporal brow incision is tied and sutured in a similar manner. The temporal rhomboid is usually not tied quite as tightly as the nasal one (Fig. 2–54). The projecting ends of the fascia are pulled with the Wright needle horizontally within the brow tract from the nasal and temporal incisions towards the middle incision. In doing this, the fascia should be inserted only 3 to 4 mm into the eye of the needle so that it will pull free deep in the tunnel as the needle is withdrawn (Fig. 2–55). If the end of the fascia still projects from the middle wound, the fascia is grasped with forceps and tension exerted on the end so that when it is cut off flush with the skin, it will retract into the incision.

Gentamycin solution is irrigated along the tracts through a blunt needle inserted in the brow incisions. The brow skin inci-

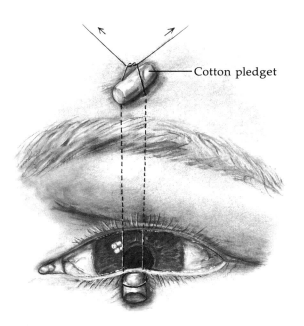

Figure 2–58 Frost suture.

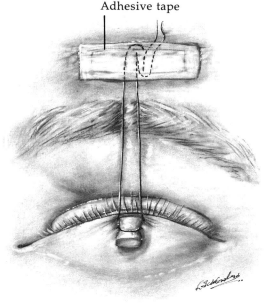

Adhesive tape

Cotton pledget

Figure 2–59 Lid closure suture.

crease or fold. The simplicity of this suture can hardly be dignified by an eponym, and it is far less severe than the original suture described by Frost.

The eye and brow are dressed with an eye pad and taped; after 24 hours, the pad and lid-closing suture are removed. A thin coating of antibiotic ointment is applied to the eye. Ointment is not used in the primary dressing as it tends to get into the wound and prevent primary closure. After 24 hours, however, ointment keeps the wound edges from crusting. The eyes are not patched after the removal of the primary dressing.

Surgery for the Correction of Jaw-Winking

If the wink is so severe that the patient and doctor elect to operate, the offending levator muscle should be transected and a bilateral frontalis sling done. Beard recommends cutting the levator in both the winking and the normal lid and then doing a bilateral sling, to give both static and dynamic symmetry. We feel this symmetry can be obtained by transecting only the abnormal levator and doing a bilateral sling.

OPERATION TO TRANSECT THE LEVATOR APONEUROSIS AND MUSCLE

General anesthesia is preferred.

The lid fold is marked by a gentle sweep of the No. 15 Bard-Parker blade across the lid in the crease. A 4–0 black silk suture is placed in the gray line, taking a firm bite. The lid plate (Storz No. SP7-13456) is covered with ointment and slipped under the lid, and the suture is fastened to the knurled knob, to put the lid on stretch. This causes a distortion of the skin and is the reason for premark-

Figures 2–60 to 2–65

Figures 2–60, 2–61 Frost suture. Severe wink reflex in adult jaw winker.
Figures 2–62 to 2–65 Postoperative—ptosis and wink are eliminated.

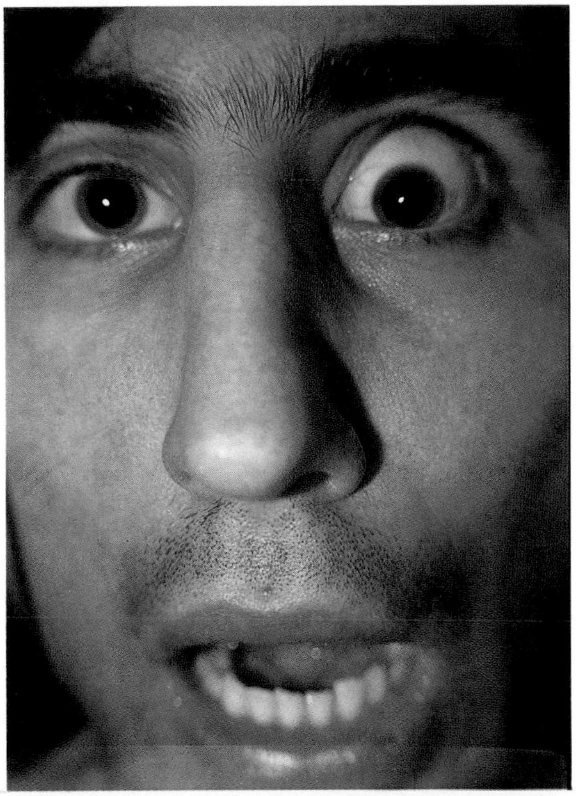

61

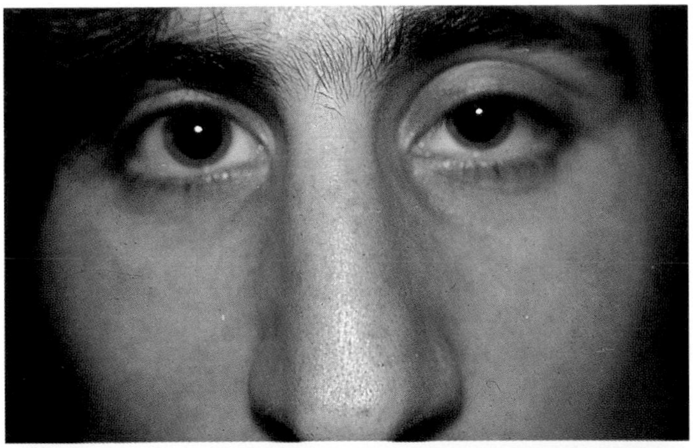

60

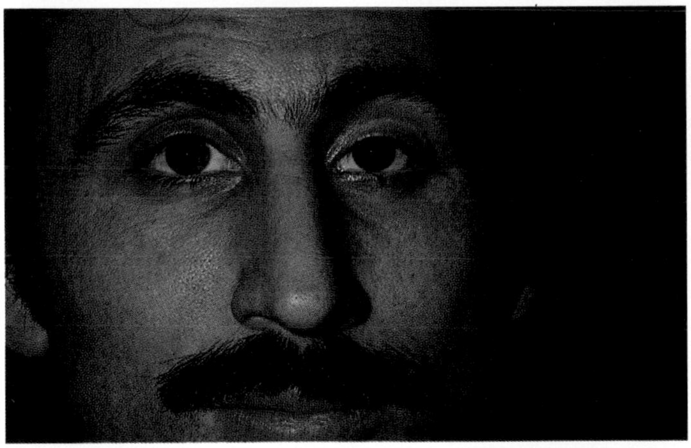

62

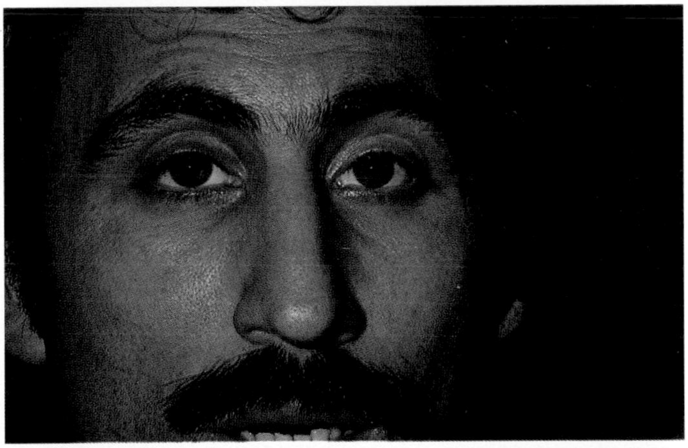

63

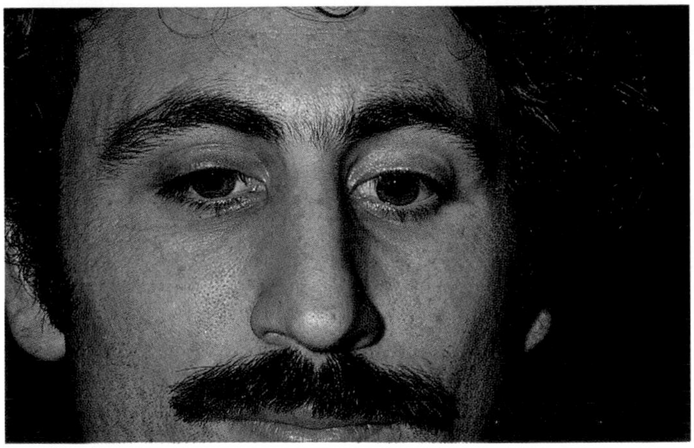

64

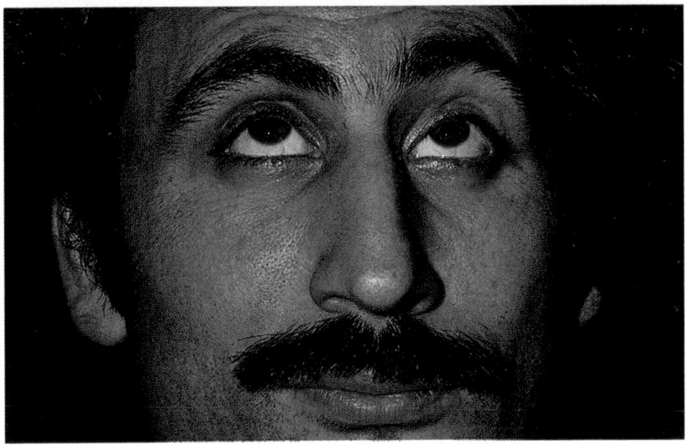

65

ing the lid fold. Scissors are used to complete the skin incision along the marked line. The subcutaneous tissue and orbicularis muscle are divided and all bleeders are occluded with cautery to give a clear view of each structure. The orbital septum is opened across the lid, and a Desmarres retractor is used to pull the upper edge of the incision towards the brow to expose the orbital fat and underlying levator aponeurosis. The dissection is carefully carried backward until the levator aponeurosis is exposed where it narrows and blends into the levator muscle. Muscle hooks are used to isolate the muscle from the anterior fat, the superior rectus muscle, and Whitnall's ligament. When the muscle and tendon have been completely isolated from these surrounding structures, a 1 cm removal of the aponeurosis is done, using cautery so that there will be no bleeding. The proximal part of the muscle retracts into the orbit above Whitnall's ligament.

With the lid still on stretch, the pretarsal muscle and levator aponeurosis are dissected downward to the lid margin. This tissue is excised to thin the lid, leaving only a small band of orbicularis muscle and 1 mm of levator aponeurosis at its insertion.

Attention is now turned to placing the slings. The inferior portions of the fascial rhomboids are fastened with 4–0 white silk to the pretarsal muscle and the levator aponeurosis where it inserts on the anterior inferior edge of the tarsus, but the fascia is not fastened to the tarsus itself. Fastening to the tarsus sometimes produces a separation of the lid from the globe as the frontalis contracts rather than the normal lid-follow on the upward gaze. The orbital septum is closed to this area with 7–0 chromic catgut and the skin is closed with 8–0 black silk. The lid plate is removed; the fascia is tightened by single knots at the nasal and temporal brow incisions and is fixed with 4–0 chromic catgut.

A routine frontalis sling is now done on the other eye. The elevation of the lid is carefully matched to that of the first eye. The skin of the brow incisions is closed in the usual manner, and both eyes are dressed with lid-closing sutures and a mild pressure dressing for 24 hours.

This procedure has worked well in our hands and we are indebted to Beard for the bilateral approach, although we have not followed his technique completely.

SUMMARY

The timing of surgery to correct the jaw-winking phenomenon depends on the severity of the ptosis and the extent of the excursion of the wink. If the ptosis is the primary cosmetic defect in the opinion of the patient, the parents, and the surgeon, it should be corrected by bilateral frontalis slings using fascia lata. If the wink reflex is the more severe problem (Figs. 2–60 and 2–61), correction by resection of the levator muscle on the affected side and bilateral frontalis slings should be done (Figs. 2–62 to 2–65). We have seen a moderate wink reflex spontaneously diminish or disappear as the child reached adult life. In our oculoplastic practice, we have seen few adult jaw-winkers in comparison to the number of children.

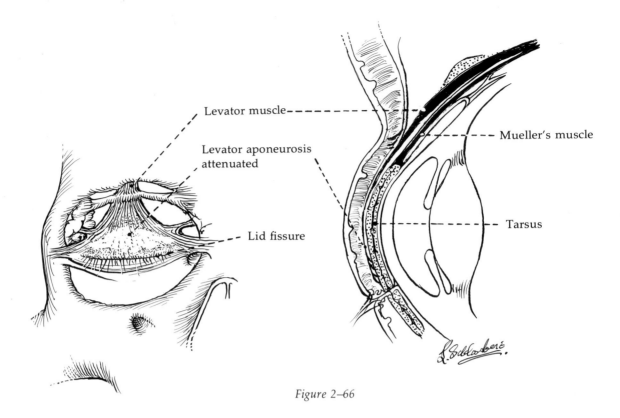

Levator muscle

Levator aponeurosis
attenuated

Lid fissure

Mueller's muscle

Tarsus

Figure 2–66

Operation: Levator Aponeurosis Resection

SMALL BLOCK RESECTION TO CORRECT
SENILE PTOSIS (Figs. 2–67 to 2–72)

The etiology and exact mechanism of senile ptosis were obscure until Jones and Quickert demonstrated dehiscences in the levator aponeurosis. Their dissection showed a thinning and in some instances partial separation of the aponeurosis above the upper edge of the tarsus (Fig. 2–66), where it normally fuses with the orbital septum.

Jones and Quickert used the obvious surgical procedure to correct this condition. Using the skin approach, they isolated the dehisced or thinned area of the aponeurosis and did an imbricating procedure, bringing sound aponeurosis from above and fastening it with buried interrupted sutures to the original insertion on the anterior surface of the tarsus. The reported results were excellent. However, when we tried their procedure we encountered difficulty in locating the attenuated aponeurosis. We found that a modification of the small block resection that we had been using for congenital ptosis patients was easier to do and gave excellent results.

The operation was planned to resect conjunctiva, Mueller's muscle, and the dehisced aponeurosis *en bloc* and to resuture the proximal components to their original insertions. This is done by putting the levator aponeurosis and Mueller's muscle on stretch with tension sutures. While traction is maintained on the tension sutures, three temporary holding sutures are placed through all thicknesses of the folded lid, to hold the tissue in place while the *en bloc*

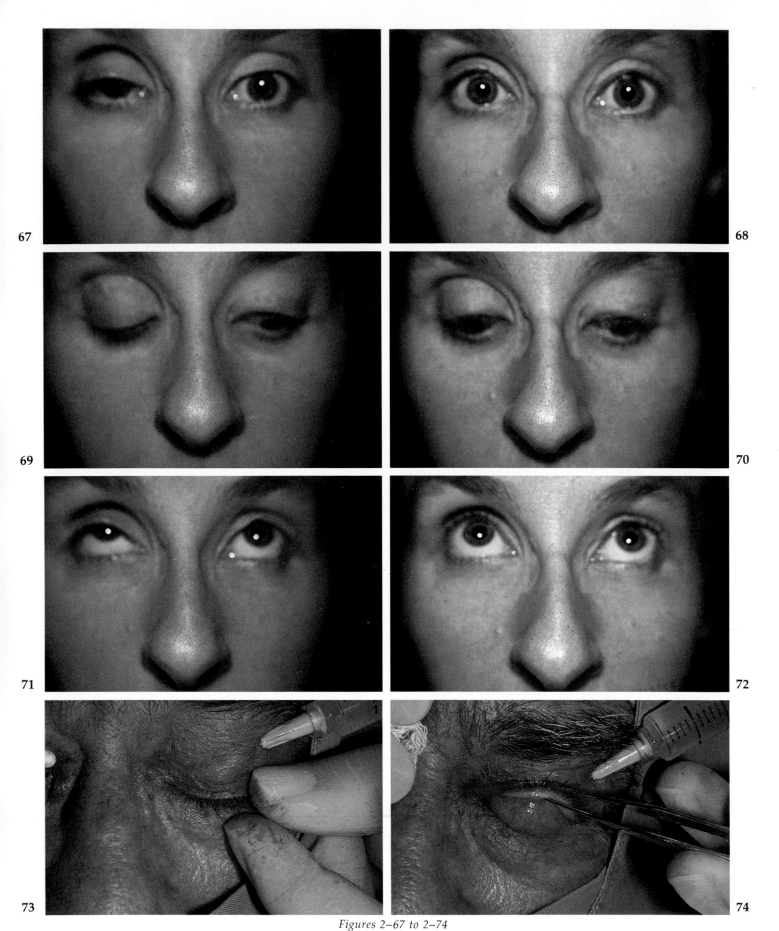

67

68

69

70

71

72

73

74

Figures 2–67 to 2–74

Figures 2–67 to 2–72   Senile ptosis, right eye; preoperative: Figs. 2–67, 2–69, 2–71;
postoperative: Figs. 2–68, 2–70, 2–72.
Figures 2–73, 2–74   Local anesthesia is used in adults.

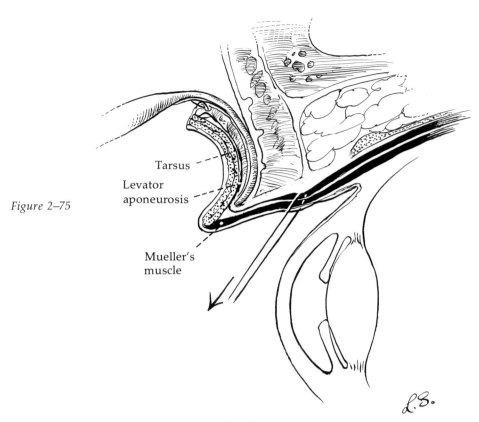

Tarsus

Levator
aponeurosis

Figure 2–75

Mueller's
muscle

resection is done, and the cut edges of the aponeurosis and Mueller's
muscle are reapproximated.

OPERATIVE TECHNIQUE

In most cases local anesthesia is used. One cc of 1 per cent
Xylocaine is injected subcutaneously across the lid with a 30-gauge
needle, beginning temporally (Fig. 2–73). Without withdrawing the
needle, the lid is everted and another 1 cc of Xylocaine is injected
to balloon the conjunctiva on the retrotarsal area (Fig. 2–74). In all
ptosis surgery, it is essential that the cornea be protected. We apply
ophthalmic ointment throughout the procedure.

The lid is everted on a Desmarres retractor, throwing the retrotarsal margin into prominence and placing the conjunctiva to the
upper fornix on stretch. Two 4–0 black silk tension sutures are
placed in the levator aponeurosis, and traction is applied to these
sutures to put the levator on stretch (Fig. 2–75). To place these sutures, a firm bite of conjunctiva, Mueller's muscle, and levator
aponeurosis is taken with Adson skin forceps 5 mm behind the
retrotarsal margin. One suture is placed at the temporal third and
one at the nasal third of the lid (Fig. 2–76). The Desmarres retractor
is removed and tension put on the sutures, which pulls the conjunctiva, Mueller's muscle, and the aponeurosis beyond the retrotarsal margin. If the pull on these sutures is transmitted to the brow
when tested by a finger in the upper sulcus, the suture is too deep
and has caught the septum and must be relocated more superficially. If the pull is transmitted back into the orbit, the aponeurosis
has been caught and the suture is in the correct plane. Nasal and

5.0 mm

63

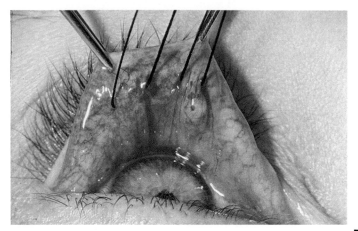

76

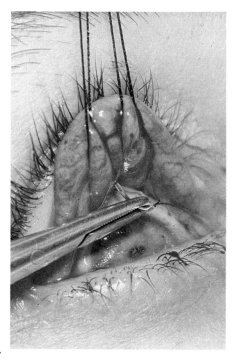

77

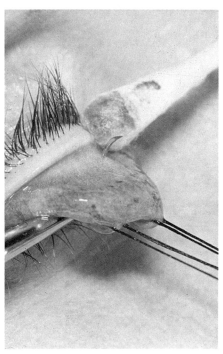

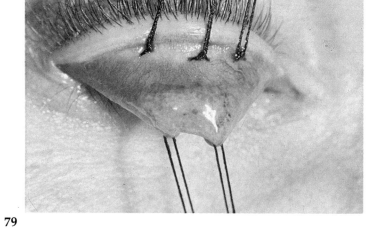

78   **79**

Figures 2–76 to 2–79

Figure 2–76   Forceps demonstrate the position of the retrotarsal margin.
Figures 2–77 to 2–79   Placement of mattress holding sutures.

lateral horns are thrown into relief and can be felt through the skin as bands going to their insertions.

While tension is exerted on these traction sutures, three double-armed 4–0 black silk temporary holding sutures are placed as a mattress stitch. The function of these sutures is to hold all the tissues of the everted lid in place after the *en bloc* resection has been done, until the proximal and distal cut edges of the aponeurosis, Mueller's muscle, and conjunctiva can be rejoined. The first holding suture is placed by passing the needle through the center of the folded lid, entering the conjunctiva 1 cm behind the tension sutures (Fig. 2–77) and emerging from tarsus and conjunctiva 1 mm from the lid edge (Fig. 2–78). The second arm of the holding suture is passed in the same way 2 mm from the first and the ends tied with a double throw surgeon's knot. The temporal and nasal holding sutures are made exactly the same way (Fig. 2–79).

1.0 CM.

Traction is put on the tension sutures, and 5 mm of the folded conjunctiva, Mueller's muscle, and aponeurosis is excised with scissors at the retrotarsal margin (Figs. 2–80 and 2–84). Since the tension sutures are placed behind the dehisced area, a firm proximal piece of aponeurosis is available to suture to the distal end at its insertion. A dry field is important; arterial bleeding from the peripheral arcade and the venous ooze are cauterized. The lid tissues, held in the folded position by the sutures, are identified from posterior to anterior as (1) conjunctiva, closely joined by (2) the rather soft Mueller's muscle, (3) the cut edge of the firmer, proximal aponeurosis, (4) the distal cut edge of the aponeurosis fastened to its insertion on the anterior lower third of the tarsus, and finally (5) the tarsus and conjunctiva (Fig. 2–81). If the scissors cut is irregular, it may be necessary to trim the edges further to given even suturing margins.

5.0 mm

A 6–0 double-armed chromic catgut suture is used to reapproximate the cut edges of the wound: one arm for the levator aponeurosis and one arm for Mueller's muscle and conjunctiva. A deep bite is taken at the right end of the incision line (the left end of the incision if the surgeon is left-handed), and a simple square knot is tied in the center of the suture (Fig. 2–85). One arm of the suture is passed across the lid for the extent of the incision using a running stitch and taking small bites (1 to 2 mm) of the proximal and distal edges of the resected levator aponeurosis, which can be identified as the firm tissue held tightly in the holding sutures (Fig. 2–82). The second arm of the suture is used in the same way to join the posterior edges of the resected Mueller's muscle and conjunctiva to their original insertions on the anterior retrotarsal margin (Fig. 2–86), catching Mueller's muscle with each bite and the conjunctiva with every second bite (Fig. 2–83). In this way, fewer loops of the suture are exposed. When the left end of the incision is reached, the two arms of the suture are tied with a square knot, and the needles are passed deep into the wound through the total thickness of the lid and brought out on the skin surface. The sutures are cut level with the skin and the ends retract into the lid tissue where they cannot rub on the cornea.

6/0 CHROMIC

The three holding sutures are cut by placing the tip of the sharp-

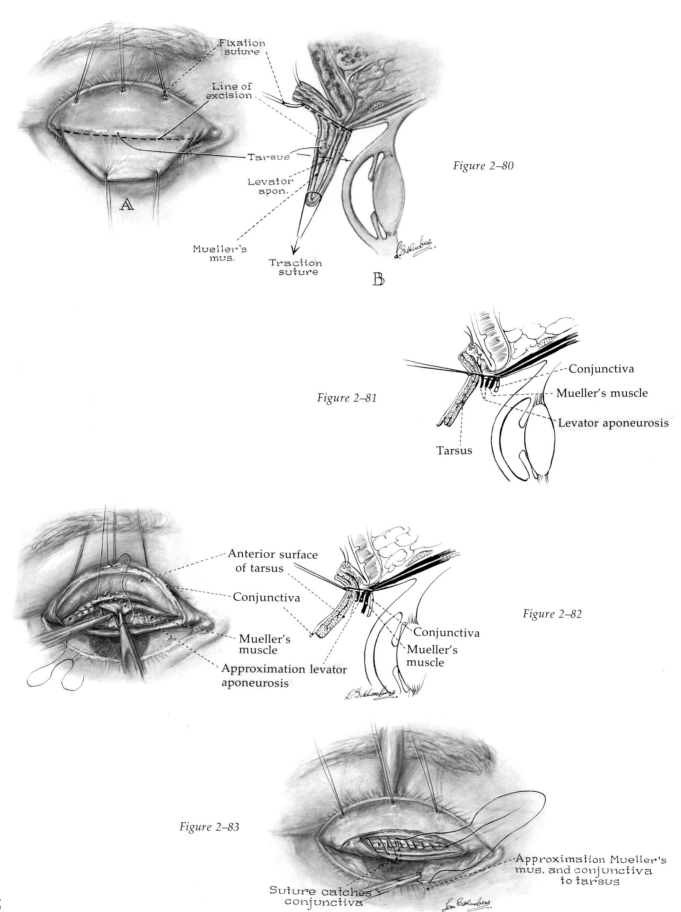

Fixation suture

Line of excision

Tarsus

Levator apon.

Mueller's mus.

Traction suture

A

B

Figure 2–80

Conjunctiva

Mueller's muscle

Levator aponeurosis

Tarsus

Figure 2–81

Anterior surface of tarsus

Conjunctiva

Mueller's muscle

Approximation levator aponeurosis

Conjunctiva

Mueller's muscle

Figure 2–82

Figure 2–83

Suture catches conjunctiva

Approximation Mueller's mus. and conjunctiva to tarsus

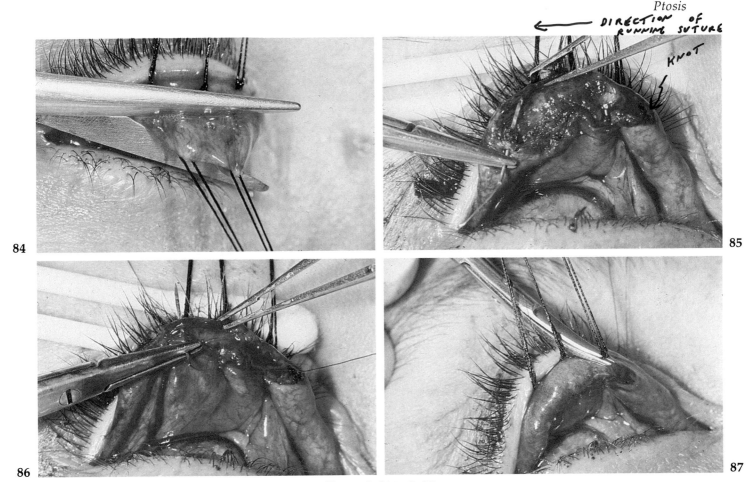

Figures 2–84 to 2–87

Figure 2–84 Block resection.
Figure 2–85 First arm of suture reapproximates levator tendon.
Figure 2–86 Second arm of suture reattaches conjunctiva and Mueller's muscle to the retrotarsal margin.
Figure 2–87 Holding sutures removed.

pointed iris scissors beneath the ties and cutting one arm of the suture so that it is completely removed (Fig. 2–87). The lid now reverts to its normal position. The eye is dressed with an eye pad in such a way that the upper lid and lashes are supported.

The eye pad is removed in 24 hours, and the patient is discharged. Antibiotic ointment is prescribed for use at night, and the lids should be closed with clear tape during sleep. The patient is instructed to apply the tape while standing before a mirror. The tape is fastened to the lower lid first and the lower lid is pulled up (rather than the upper lid down) and fastened to the brow. No eye pad is used because during sleep the lids often come open and pressure of the pad against the pillow rubs the cornea. The tape is smooth and does not stick to the damp cornea, so if the lids do come open, no damage results.

ADVANTAGES OF SMALL BLOCK RESECTION

The small block resection does not damage the tarsus, so there is less likelihood of producing a tented or peaked lid margin. The glands are not disturbed. The pull of the levator aponeurosis refastened to its original insertion turns the lashes slightly upward and outward into

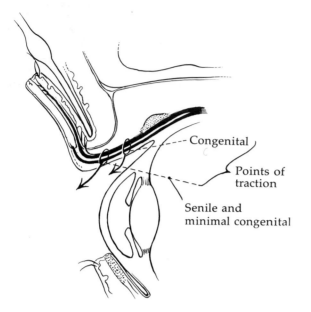

--- Congenital

Points of traction

Senile and minimal congenital

Figure 2–88 Placement of traction sutures differs for senile and minimal congenital, and congenital ptosis.

their normal position. We feel that the dehiscences of the levator aponeurosis are repaired most easily by this method.

SMALL BLOCK RESECTION TO CORRECT MILD CONGENITAL PTOSIS (Figs. 2–89 and 2–90)

A mild congenital ptosis (1 to 2 mm) usually has a good amplitude of contraction (8+ mm) and an excellent lid fold. Preoperatively, we would estimate that it needs a 10 to 12 mm resection of the aponeurosis.

In congenital ptosis, where there should be interdigitating muscle fibers at the junction between the aponeurosis and muscle, fewer and fewer muscle fibers appear, according to the severity of the ptosis. In essence, we are dealing with a longer aponeurosis, or tendon, with a proportional lessening of the contractibility of the shortened muscle. (In the senile ptosis, the thinning or dehiscence of the aponeurosis has separated the normal muscle contraction from the lid.) The small block resection removes 10 to 12 mm of the over-long tendon, thus allowing the muscle that remains to raise the lid higher.

The operative procedure is exactly the same as described for senile ptosis. As at the end of any congenital ptosis procedure, a lid-closing suture is necessary to support the upper lid and protect the cornea in the initial postoperative period (Fig. 2–91). One or two sutures are placed in the lower lid and fastened to adhesive tape on the brow to effectively close the lid (see p. 58). The eye pad and lid-closing suture are removed in 24 hours, and the patient is discharged from the hospital. Antibiotic ointment and lid taping at night are used as with senile ptosis.

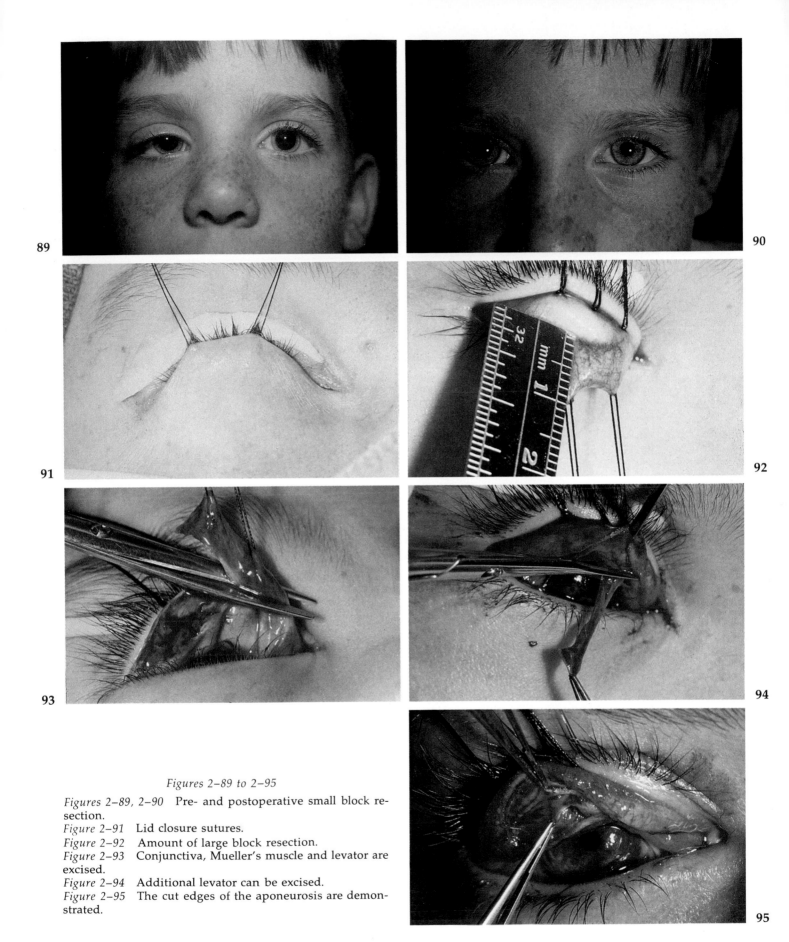

89 **90**

91 **92**

93 **94**

Figures 2–89 to 2–95

Figures 2–89, 2–90 Pre- and postoperative small block resection.
Figure 2–91 Lid closure sutures.
Figure 2–92 Amount of large block resection.
Figure 2–93 Conjunctiva, Mueller's muscle and levator are excised.
Figure 2–94 Additional levator can be excised.
Figure 2–95 The cut edges of the aponeurosis are demonstrated.

95

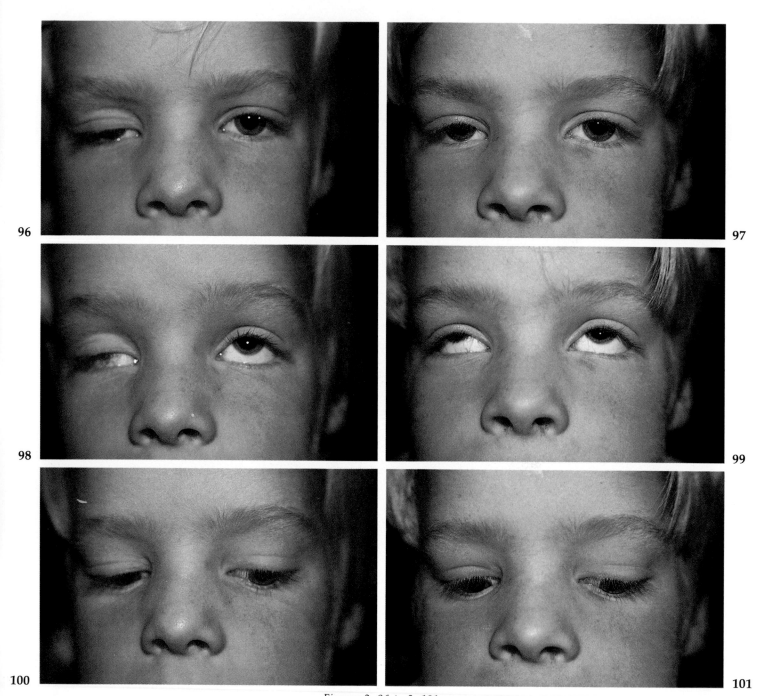

96

97

98

99

100

101

Figures 2–96 to 2–101

Figures 2–96, 2–98, 2–100   Preoperative.
Figures 2–97, 2–99, 2–101   Postoperative large block resection for severe congenital ptosis with some levator function.

LARGE BLOCK RESECTION TO CORRECT
MODERATE CONGENITAL PTOSIS

A moderate congenital ptosis (3 mm) has fair (5 to 7 mm) amplitude of function and fair or poor lid fold and requires 18 mm of aponeurosis resection.

The tension sutures are placed 1 cm behind the retrotarsal margin. When the Desmarres lid retractor everts the lid, the conjunctiva and Mueller's muscle are markedly stretched to 2.5 to 3.0 cm. The levator aponeurosis, being fibrous, does not stretch, but the levator muscle itself stretches. Thus, a resection of the aponeurosis is the actual amount of fibrous tissue caught by the tension sutures. The resection of the conjunctiva and Mueller's muscle is relative; since this tissue has been markedly stretched, the actual resection is not as great.

We have seen no ill effects nor have we noted any late-developing problems from the resection of this amount of conjunctiva, either with this procedure or the procedure described in 1954.* The block resection done at that time was with a slightly different manner of suturing.

The large block resection differs from the small block resection in two ways: (1) The traction sutures are placed 8 to 10 mm behind the retrotarsal margin (Fig. 2–88) and more traction is applied (Fig. 2–92) while the scissors cut is made (Fig. 2–93). (2) Further trimming of the proximal aponeurosis can be done after this initial cut has been made in such a way that no more of the conjunctiva and Mueller's muscle is resected (Figs. 2–94 and 2–95).

COMMENTS ON LEVATOR APONEUROSIS
RESECTIONING

In the small and large block resections, only the central portion of the aponeurosis is removed. The horns and Whitnall's ligament are not cut.

The suturing of the proximal portion of the aponeurosis to the original insertion on the anterior lower one third of the tarsus seems to account for the improved results of this method over the method we previously reported in 1954.

The resection of the conjunctiva increases the tension on the attachments to the superior rectus muscle in the upper cul-de-sac, so on upward gaze the superior rectus muscle acts as a secondary elevator of the lid. How much this actually affects the success of the operation is difficult to say, but it certainly is a plus for the procedure (Figs. 2–96 to 2–101).

Operation: Maximum Resection, with Cutting of the Horns and Whitnall's Ligament

A severe congenital ptosis (4 mm or more), with poor amplitude levator function (less than 4 mm) and little or no lid fold requires a maximum resection with cutting of the horns and Whitnall's ligament.

---

*Iliff, C. E.: A simplified ptosis operation. Am. J. Ophthal. 37:529, 1954.

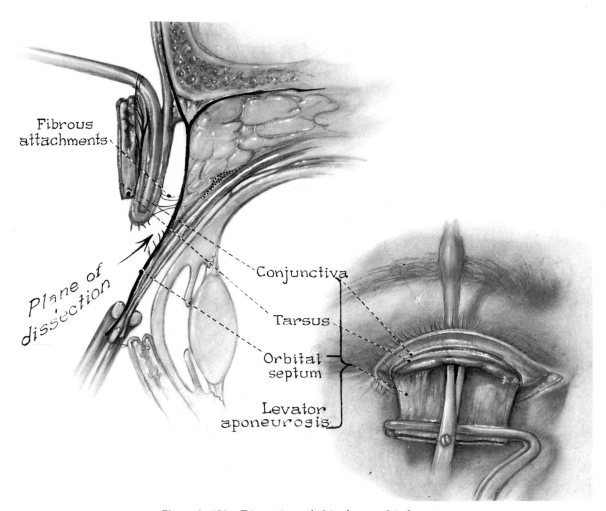

Figure 2–102 Dissection of skin from orbital septum.

The anticipated resection is 18 to 24 mm. The upper lid is everted with a Desmarres retractor. A small cut is made with scissors on the lateral side of the retrotarsal edge through the conjunctiva, Mueller's muscle, levator aponeurosis, and orbital septum into the potential space between the tarsus and the skin (Fig. 2–103). Blunt scissors are directed into this incision and with a gentle opening and closing motion are passed across the subcutaneous space immediately beneath the skin to the nasal edge of the retrotarsal margin (Fig. 2–104). The scissors tips are then spread and the conjunctiva between the scissors tips is cut with a second pair of scissors. One blade of the ptosis clamp (Storz No. E-2504) is placed between the blades of the scissors, which hold the clamp gently so that the scissors and clamp can be manipulated as one unit (Fig. 2–105). As the scissors are withdrawn, the blade of the clamp is advanced across the scissors tract, to emerge at the temporal incision. The clamp is locked; in its bite are contained conjunctiva, the superior edge of the tarsus to which Mueller's muscle is attached, the superior arcade of arteries, the aponeurosis of the levator, orbital septum, and some of the fibers of the preseptal muscle. An incision is made distal to the clamp through all the structures held by the clamp (Fig. 2–106). Bleeders are cauterized to produce a dry field.

The clamp is lifted away from the cut and everted tarsal plate, exposing the fine interdigitating fibrous attachments that extend from the levator and orbital septum to the skin to make the lid crease. These fibers are divided by blunt and sharp dissection with scissors, taking care not to buttonhole the skin, which is usually tented at the area of the fibrous attachments (Figs. 2–102 and 2–107). Dissection is extended almost to the orbital rim, and the septum is visible as a well-defined plane of tissue. The Desmarres lid retractor is removed and the orbital septum cut free from the clamp. A tug on the septum with toothed forceps is transmitted to the brow (Fig. 2–108). A pull on the levator clamp is transmitted directly back into the orbit. The septum is then separated from the aponeurosis (Fig. 2–109). Traction on the clamp, which is holding the central portion of the levator aponeurosis, throws the lateral and nasal horns of the aponeurosis into relief. These are cut with scissors; the scissors are directed vertically along the edges of the tendon to prevent damage to the superior oblique tendon or the lacrimal gland (Fig. 2–111). The orbital septum is retracted upward with the Desmarres retractor, and tension is placed on the levator clamp so that blunt dissection can be carried out to expose orbital fat, an important landmark between the septum and the tendon. The fat and the septum are caught beneath the Desmarres retractor, and Whitnall's ligament is brought into view. This transverse ligament is an extension of the levator capsule, extending nasally to the area of the trochlea and temporally to the fascia of the lacrimal gland. If tight, the ligament should be incised by making a vertical cut on each side of the levator tendon. Tension is put on the levator clamp and the conjunctiva is incised at 1 mm proximal to the clamp and can be easily freed backward for at least 1 cm toward the upper cul-de-sac.

Three double-armed 4–0 black silk holding mattress sutures are then placed through the levator aponeurosis 2 mm above the desired

Text continued on page 78

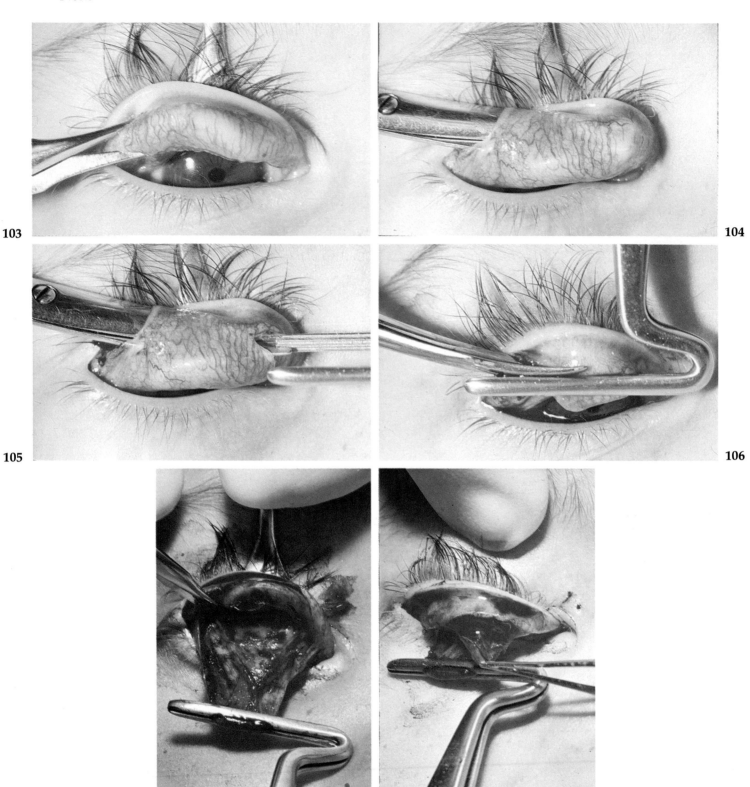

103

104

105

106

107

108

Figures 2–103 to 2–108

Figure 2–103 Buttonhole conjunctiva at retrotarsal edge.
Figure 2–104 Scissors are passed in subcutaneous potential space.
Figure 2–105 Grasping ptosis clamp with scissors facilitates its passage.
Figure 2–106 Cut distal to clamp.
Figure 2–107 Dissection is carried between skin and septum.
Figure 2–108 Pull on forceps identifies orbital septum.

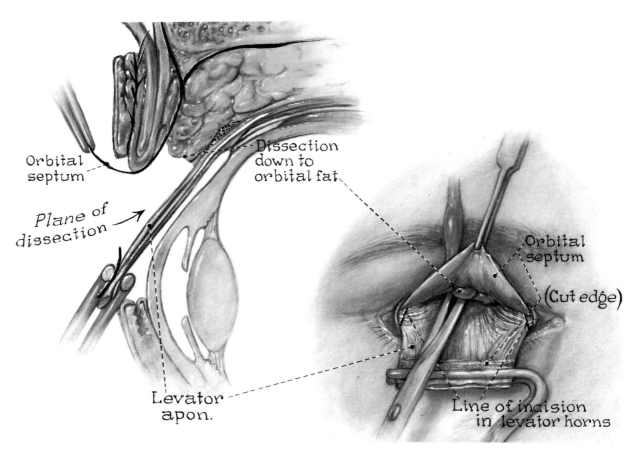

Figure 2–109   The orbital septum is separated from the aponeurosis.

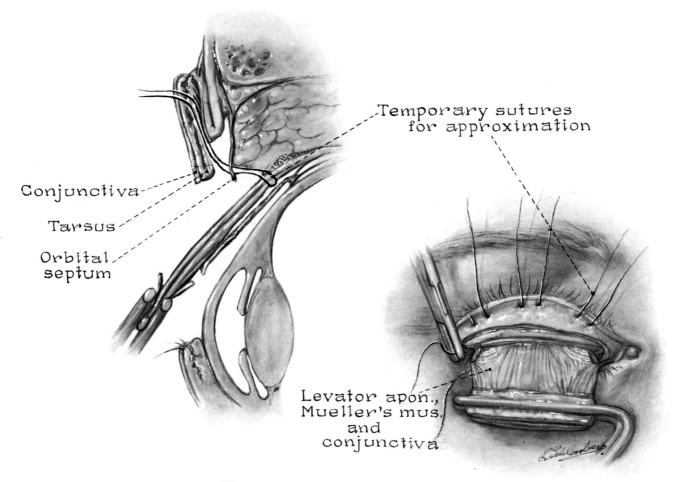

Temporary sutures
for approximation

Conjunctiva

Tarsus

Orbital
septum

Levator apon.,
Mueller's mus.
and
conjunctiva

Figure 2–110   Placement of holding sutures.

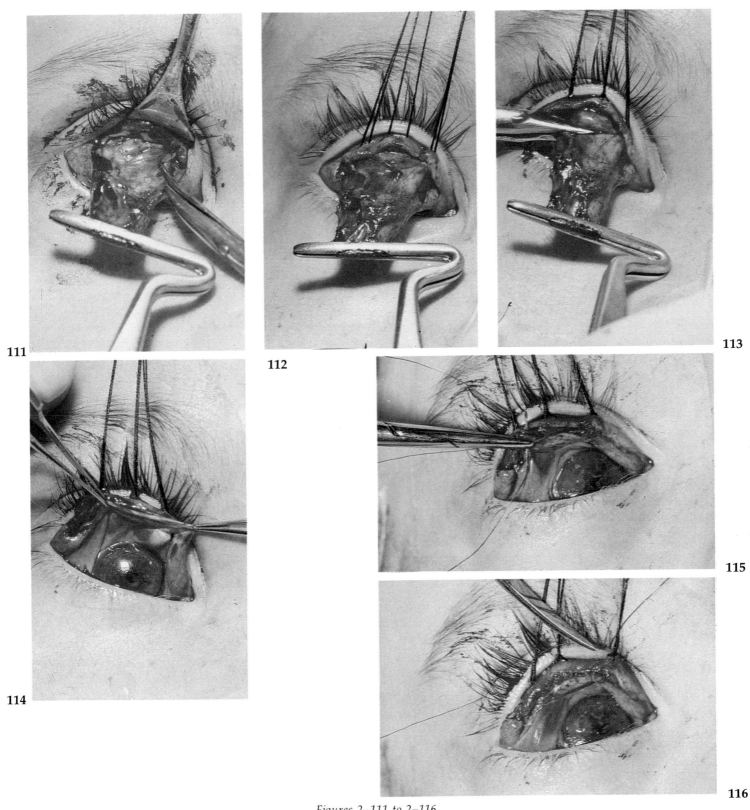

111

112

113

114

115

116

Figures 2–111 to 2–116

Figure 2–111   Horns are cut.
Figure 2–112   Holding sutures placed.
Figure 2–113   Cut 2 mm. distal to holding sutures.
Figure 2–114   Conjunctiva preserved.
Figure 2–115   Levator is reattached to tarsus.
Figure 2–116   Mueller's muscle and conjunctiva are sutured to tarsus—holding sutures
are cut out.

level of resection (20 to 22 mm from the cut tarsal edge) and brought out through the everted tarsus 1 mm from the lid margin (Figs. 2–110 and 2–112). The two arms of the suture are tied with a double surgeon's knot. These holding sutures will keep the aponeurosis and the tarsus in that position.

The aponeurosis is excised 2 mm distal to the preplaced holding sutures (Figs. 2–113 and 2–114). Since the ptosis clamp was placed originally at the upper margin of the tarsus, approximately 3 mm of the levator aponeurosis was left attached to the insertion. Therefore, if a resection of 18 mm is done, the cut edge is advanced to the original insertion, and an effective 21 mm of resection will be accomplished. A double-armed 6–0 chromic catgut suture is used to reapproximate the aponeurosis in exactly the same manner as was done in a small block resection for senile ptosis (Fig. 2–115). Conjunctiva and Mueller's muscle are reattached to the retrotarsal margin as was described (Figs. 2–116 to 2–119).

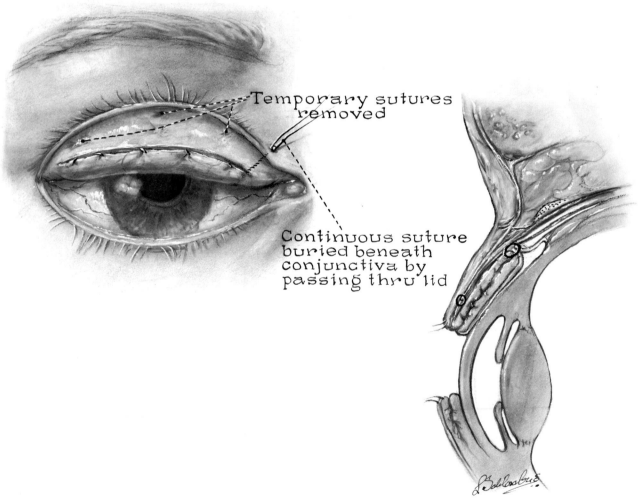

Figure 2–117   Position of running sutures.

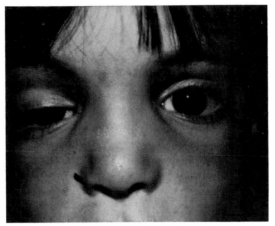

Figure 2–118 Preoperative.

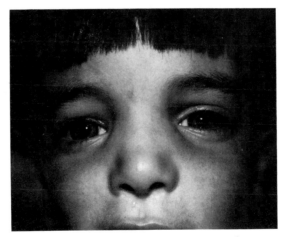

Figure 2–119 Postoperative—maximum levator resection for severe congenital ptosis (little levator function).

Operation: Levator Resection — Skin Approach

We have rarely used the skin approach made popular by Berke* (Fig. 2–120), except in patients in whom the ptosis was accompanied by some conjunctival pathology (scarring, papilloma, vernal conjunctivitis, or a ptosis iatrogenically produced by overenergetic dissection of a conjunctival tumor) or in patients in whom a ptosis procedure by the conjunctival route failed. After an unsuccessful procedure, it is better to enter the lid through a new site above the scarred area of the previous incision.

With this technique, the lateral and nasal horns and the transverse ligament can be cut and the levator tendon shortened and advanced. A lid crease is established by a second row of sutures.

The skin, subcutaneous tissue, and orbicularis muscle are incised at the level of the skin crease (premarked with a No. 15 Bard-Parker knife) to expose the orbital septum. Dissection is carried down at this plane almost to the lashline, and upward for approximately 1 cm.

The septum is then divided with a horizontal incision to free it from the tarsus, and the dissection is carried superiorly and posteriorly to expose the orbital fat, which is a landmark separating the septum from the levator tendon. The upper skin flap and septum are retracted upward; the levator aponeurosis and conjunctiva are buttonholed 25 mm apart at the retrotarsal margin, and a ptosis clamp is applied. A horizontal incision is made through all these structures distal to the ptosis clamp at the upper edge of the tarsus. Upward tension is put on the ptosis clamp, and Wescott scissors are used to dissect the conjunctiva from Mueller's muscle as far back as the fornix. The conjunctiva is cut free along the edge of the ptosis clamp, leaving Mueller's muscle and the levator aponeurosis in the bite of the clamp.

The conjunctiva is resutured to the upper edge of the tarsus with 7–0 chromic catgut. This fine suture must be carefully buried in the lid tissue so it does not rub on the cornea. The reason for making the incision through the conjunctiva and resuturing it to its original position is that it is extremely difficult to dissect the conjunctiva from Mueller's muscle unless it is mobilized by putting it on stretch with the clamp.

Tension is put on the levator tendon and Mueller's muscle by pulling on the ptosis clamp so that the horns can be put on stretch and divided. Whitnall's ligament, the check ligament of the levator, is identified and divided nasally and temporally if it interferes with the movement of the levator. (Care must be taken to avoid damaging the tendon of the superior oblique muscle, which passes nasally just under Whitnall's ligament.) The upper lid is elevated manually to 2 mm below the upper limbus with the eye in the primary position. Then, with moderate tension on the ptosis clamp to put the levator on stretch, one 4–0 plain double-armed catgut suture is placed through the tendon at the level of the lid margin and is tied to include the

*Berke, R. N.: Results of resection of the levator muscle through a skin incision in congenital ptosis. Arch. Ophthalmol., 62:177, 1959.

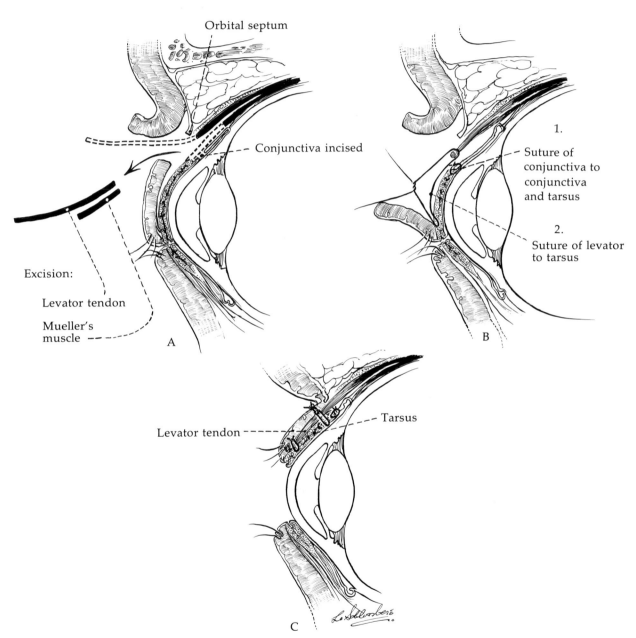

Figure 2–120 Anterior approach for levator resection.

central one third of the tendon (or muscle, depending on the amount of the proposed resection). The amount of tendon that can be resected ranges from 8 to 25 mm. In most instances, we consider the preoperative measurements and, in addition, check the amount of resection indicated by pulling the tendon down over the lid while the lid is held at the desired level. Two similar double-armed sutures are placed on either side of the central suture and are tied to catch the nasal and lateral thirds of the tendon, which is then excised 3 mm anterior to the three tied sutures. One arm of each of these sutures is passed through the superficial layer of the tarsus just posterior to the lash line and is tied, advancing the tendon onto the lower anterior tarsal surface.

Three double-armed 4–0 plain catgut sutures are passed through the lid from the conjunctival surface at the level of the upper tarsal edge, to fix the advanced levator tendon. One arm of the suture passes through the upper skin flap and one through the lower so that when they are tied a lid crease is created.

The lower lid is fastened to adhesive tape on the brow with a 6–0 black silk suture for corneal protection for 24 hours. Since this operation has been so well described by Berke and others,* we feel it unnecessary to illustrate it in detail here (Figs. 2–121 and 2–122).

---

*Fox, S. A.: *Surgery of Ptosis.* Grune & Stratton, New York, 1968. Callahan, A.: *Surgery of the Eye.* Charles C Thomas, Springfield, Ill., 1956. Beard, C.: *Ptosis.* C. V. Mosby, St Louis, 1976.

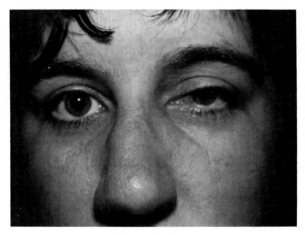

Figure 2–121

Ptosis following conjunctival surgery for acquired melanosis.

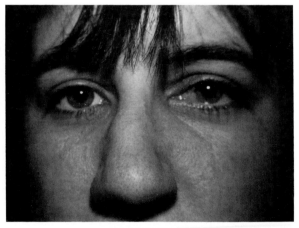

Figure 2–122

Postoperative—ptosis correction by skin approach.

Lower Lid Ptosis

In some children in addition to the ptosis of the upper lid, there is a ptosis of the lateral half of the lower lid. This is apparent preoperatively, but postoperatively it would become a rather glaring defect.

The correction depends on whether the ptosis is caused by tight skin and subcutaneous tissue pulling the lid down — similar to a cicatricial ectropion — or by a loss of substance of the tarsus, which makes the supporting tissue deficient.

If the skin is tight, it is possible to rotate a tongue of skin and orbicularis muscle from the upper lid to relieve the tension. This will permit a nice lid crease to be made in the upper lid, and with the tongue of tissue fastened temporally, will bolster up the tight ptosed lower lid.

On the other hand, if the tarsus — the skeleton of the lower lid — is deficient, it is possible to fill in the defect by transplanting tarsus from the retrotarsal area of the upper lid at the time of the ptosis procedure on that lid. This tarsal-conjunctival free graft usually takes well and gives excellent support to the lateral half of the lid.

COMPLICATIONS OF PTOSIS SURGERY

The complications of ptosis surgery include undercorrection, poor lid crease, overcorrection, peaked lid, infection, corneal staining, ectropion, entropion, and loss of lashes.

Undercorrection

Undercorrection is a complication encountered more frequently in surgery for congenital ptosis. It occurs when not enough aponeurosis and levator are resected; when tight horns or Whitnall's check ligaments are not recognized as limiting the muscle action and are not cut; or when all the tissues are so abnormal that only partial correction can be obtained. The patient and the patient's family must understand that the surgeon cannot remake completely what has been a failure in development. In some cases, it is impossible to achieve a perfect result. When an undercorrection does occur and the patient and surgeon feel that further surgery is indicated, the amount of motion should be reevaluated and surgery planned accordingly. If the ptosis is only very slight, we are inclined to repeat the procedure and resect 2 to 3 mm of tarsus with a block resection. On the other hand, if very little improvement has been obtained with the first procedure, we will use a skin approach to attack the aponeurosis and tendon above the site of previous surgery. In this way we encounter less bleeding, and the aponeurosis is much more easily identified.

Poor Lid Crease

A poor lid crease postoperatively can be corrected by making an incision through the skin where the lid fold should be.

Since methylene blue or other marking inks smear or become indistinct when the lid is put on stretch, distorting the usual crease line, we routinely mark the lid crease with a light incision. If a crease is indistinct, the lid edge is pushed upward a number of times with a cotton swab to produce a natural crease in the skin. With the lid pushed up, a No. 15 Bard-Parker knife is passed very lightly across the lid in the crease to mark the skin. This cut will remain when the lid is put on stretch and will indicate where the incision is to be made to make a lid crease or for the anterior approach for levator shortening.

A 4–0 black silk suture is placed in the gray line and tied to the knurled knob on the lid plate to put the lid on a mild stretch. The skin is incised along the marked crease with sharp-pointed iris scissors. Bleeding is controlled with cautery. The incision is carried down through the orbicularis to the orbital septum. If the skin is redundant, an elliptical section can be removed with scissors (Fig. 2–123). A 7–0 chromic catgut suture is used to invaginate the skin edges and fasten them to the orbital septum to make a lid crease. The needle is passed through the orbital septum and levator aponeurosis, taking a small bite of tissue, and then passed through the upper skin edge and the lower skin edge. A tie is made deep in the incision, the knot being completely buried (Fig. 2–124). Occasionally at the time of surgery, the lid crease does not seem to extend as far nasally or temporally as desirable and this method is used to extend it. This has proven most effective in our hands and has been better than through-and-through lid sutures. A lid closure suture and tape to the brow is used (Figs. 2–125 to 2–128).

Overcorrection

Overcorrection in congenital ptosis is unusual but does occur if a suture is inadvertently placed through Whitnall's ligament during a resection of the aponeurosis, fastening the lid to the firm fascia of the brow. Correction requires taking the wound down and cutting the offending suture (Figs. 2–129 and 2–130).

Overcorrection, if it is very slight, should be treated with massage for 2 to 3 months. If slight overcorrection remains, Berke's tarso-aponeurosis tenotomy through the tarsal plate gives good results. It consists of everting the lid on a Desmarres retractor and making an incision through the tarsus approximately 2 mm from

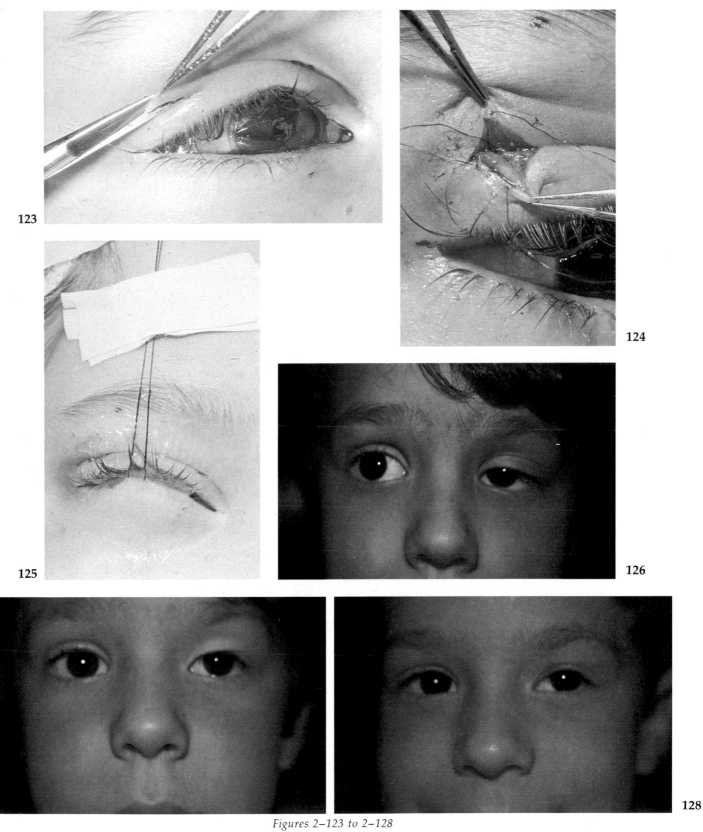

Figures 2–123 to 2–128

Figures 2–123 to 2–125   Creation of lid fold.
Figure 2–126   Preoperative ptosis.
Figure 2–127   Postoperative ptosis procedure—no lid fold.
Figure 2–128   Postoperative creation of lid fold.

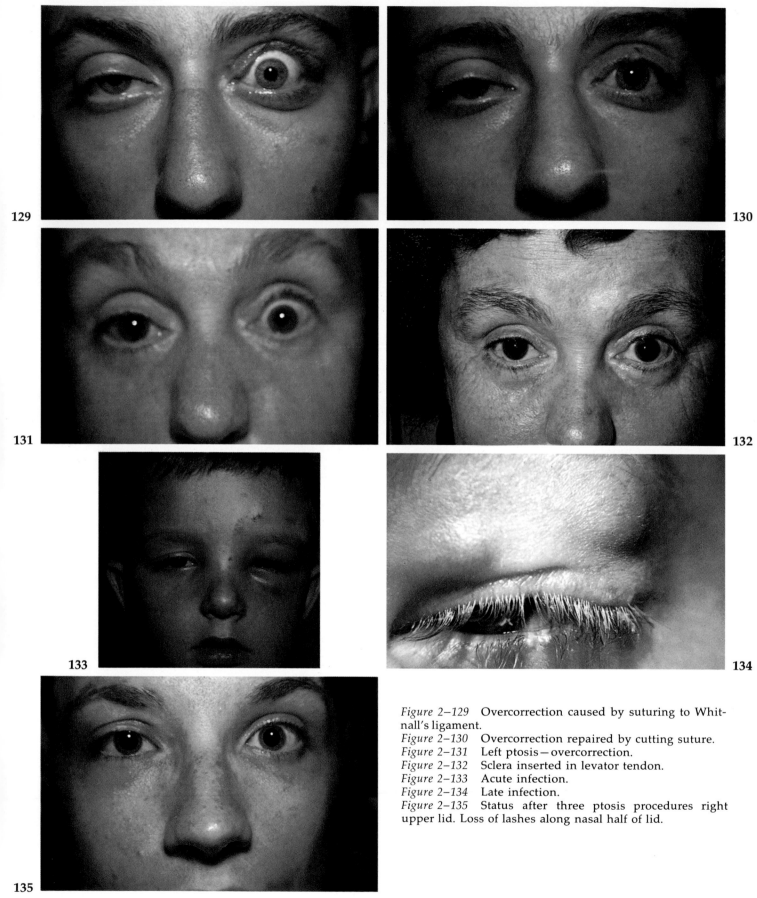

Figure 2–129 Overcorrection caused by suturing to Whitnall's ligament.
Figure 2–130 Overcorrection repaired by cutting suture.
Figure 2–131 Left ptosis—overcorrection.
Figure 2–132 Sclera inserted in levator tendon.
Figure 2–133 Acute infection.
Figure 2–134 Late infection.
Figure 2–135 Status after three ptosis procedures right upper lid. Loss of lashes along nasal half of lid.

Figures 2–129 to 2–135

the retrotarsal margin, through conjunctiva, tarsus, levator aponeurosis, and orbital septum, leaving only the skin. This incision is across the whole tarsus. An inverted Frost suture from the upper lid to the lower lid is used, and the suture is taped to the cheek to apply mild traction downward for 8 to 10 days. Although minor overcorrection can be reversed this way, there may be considerable discomfort and occasional tissue reaction from the Frost suture, and therefore, the suture may have to be removed sooner.

If an overcorrection is noted in the first few days after a small block or large block resection, it is possible to do a Berke's tarso-aponeurosis tenotomy immediately by cutting the tarsus below the suture line. If this does not reverse the overcorrection, a piece of sclera will ultimately have to be placed in the levator tendon where it narrows to join the levator muscle (Figs. 2–131 and 2–132).

INSERTION OF SCLERA INTO APONEUROSIS

General anesthesia should be used, as local anesthesia distorts the tissues and makes the dissection difficult. The anterior approach is made as previously described — through the lid fold, the orbicularis, and orbital septum. These are retracted upward with a Desmarres retractor, and the levator tendon and muscle are isolated.

A piece of preserved sclera the width of the muscle is inserted. The length of the sclera should be three times the amount of overcorrection plus 2 mm, assuming that 1 mm will be caught in the suture line at each end of the anastomosis. For example, if the lid is 2 mm too high, an 8 mm [(2 mm $\times$ 3) + 2 mm] piece of sclera will be needed to drop the lid to the desired position.

Suturing to each end of the lengthened muscle is done by a mattress stitch with 6–0 chromic catgut. The orbital septum is not resutured, but the skin is closed with closely spaced 8–0 black silk sutures. Decadron is injected beneath the suture line, and a firm pressure bandage is applied. The eye is kept bandaged with mild pressure for 1 week.

Grafts of sclera at the upper edge of the tarsus, either buried under the conjunctiva or left bare, have not given us as consistently good results as the grafts at the tendon-muscle junction. However, if overcorrection is markedly nasal or temporal, attention has to be directed to this particular area, especially if the exact course of the previous surgery is not known. In this case, the sclera is inserted either temporally or nasally beneath the conjunctiva at the upper edge of the tarsus.

Peaked Lid

After a Frontalis Sling. If at the time of surgery one arm of the sling is too tight, it will produce a peaking of the lid, which usually can be relieved by grasping the lid margin at the site of the peak by Adson forceps and pulling with a see-saw motion to reset the arms of the rhomboid. If this maneuver is not sufficient, the knot of

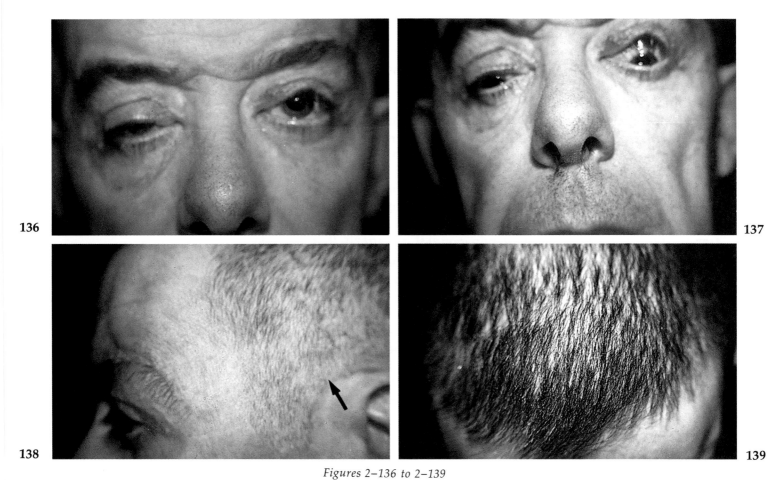

Figures 2–136 to 2–139

Figures 2–136, 2–137 Left upper lid immobile and peaked, cornea stained diffusely.
Figures 2–138, 2–139 Incision was carried across the scalp.

Oddities

Occasionally, bizarre ptosis procedures with disastrous results are encountered. Figures 2–136 to 2–139 show a patient with marked overcorrection from sling procedures performed through an incision from ear to ear over the top of the head. The fascia was led to silver wires emerging at the incision which were tightened on the third postoperative day to further elevate the lids. An overcorrection occurred; the patient was unable to close the left eye and lost some vision because of corneal drying. Correction was accomplished by cutting the fascial slings.

POSTOPERATIVE CARE FOR ALL PTOSIS PROCEDURES

Day Patching

In children, if only one eye is operated upon, it has been found beneficial to patch the *unoperated* eye during the day. The normal postoperative reaction to any surgical procedure on an eye is to close the lid. The orbicularis muscle is so much more powerful than any of the levators that this closure is often quite forceful and puts a strain on the suture line of the newly shortened tendon. If the unoperated eye is patched, the patient tends to hold the operated eye open and, because it is painful, closes it less forcefully in blinking. The unoperated eye is usually patched for three to four days.

Night Patching

Postoperative closure of the operated eye (or eyes) at night with clear plastic tape for two to three weeks is helpful in avoiding corneal irritation. One inch wide tape is used and is stuck firmly to the lower lid and cheek and pulled upward to adhere to the brow. It is a substitute for a lid closing suture. No eye pad is used for two reasons. First, the clear tape gives the parent — if a child is being treated — a clear view and thus assurance that the lids are closed. Second, sometimes during sleep the lids come open, and the gauze pad itself may rub the cornea. The smooth plastic tape, on the other hand, will not stick to the cornea and will not cause corneal abrasion, actually acting as protection.

Restriction of activities in children is almost impossible, yet we feel a certain amount of restraint is indicated. Several patients have had the suture line broken open by a blow to the eye during friendly rough-house with siblings.

The postoperative swelling of the lid may somewhat limit the immediate evaluation of the effectiveness of the surgery, and 2 months are allowed before final evaluation.

3
Blepharoplasty

Blepharochalasis is the term used to describe a "baggy" appearance of the lids (Fig. 3–3). Relaxation of skin is the primary component, but it may be accompanied by weakness of the preseptal muscle (orbicularis) and the orbital septum, allowing protrusion of orbital fat (Figs. 3–1 and 3–2). Rarely, blepharochalasis may occur as a herniation of orbital fat through a congenital defect in the orbital septum (Fig. 3–4). It is possible for the protrusion of fat to occur in the absence of a significant sagging of the skin. A similar appearance can be produced by recurrent swelling of the lids of probable allergic etiology (Fig. 3–5), but this swelling is unlike congenital blepharochalasis in that the skin covers edematous tissue anterior to the orbital septum, not prolapsed fat. As time goes on, the recurrent allergic phenomenon causes the skin and deeper structures of the lids to become markedly relaxed and atrophic.

The term "dermachalasis of the lid" is used to describe relaxation of only the skin without any other changes in the lid (Fig. 3–6). This more specific terminology evolved to indicate the type of surgical correction required. Dermachalasis of the lid requires only the removal of skin for correction; correction of blepharochalasis is a more extensive procedure in which orbital fat is excised, the relaxed orbital septum is tightened, and in some instances the lid is thinned by the removal of hypertrophied orbicularis muscle.

Preoperative Considerations

Both dermachalasis and blepharochalasis have two aspects. The obvious one is the cosmetic blemish that is the usual concern of the patient and the reconstructive surgeon. The more important aspect is the asthenopic symptoms that are produced. The patient does not associate the symptoms with the cosmetic conditions, and frequently even the ophthalmologist fails to recognize their true etiology. The actual fatigue the patient experiences in elevating the heavy, overloaded upper lids and the unpleasant, watery, draggy feeling

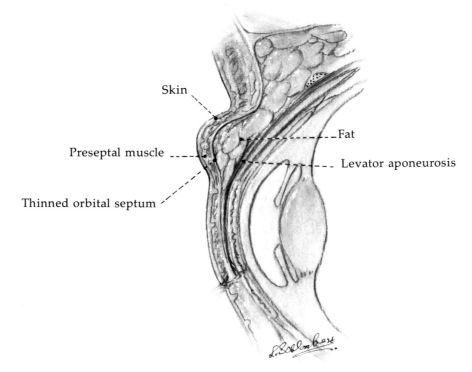

Skin

Fat

Preseptal muscle

Levator aponeurosis

Thinned orbital septum

Figure 3–1 Blepharochalasis; lax skin and weakness in orbicularis and orbital septum causing orbital fat protrusion.

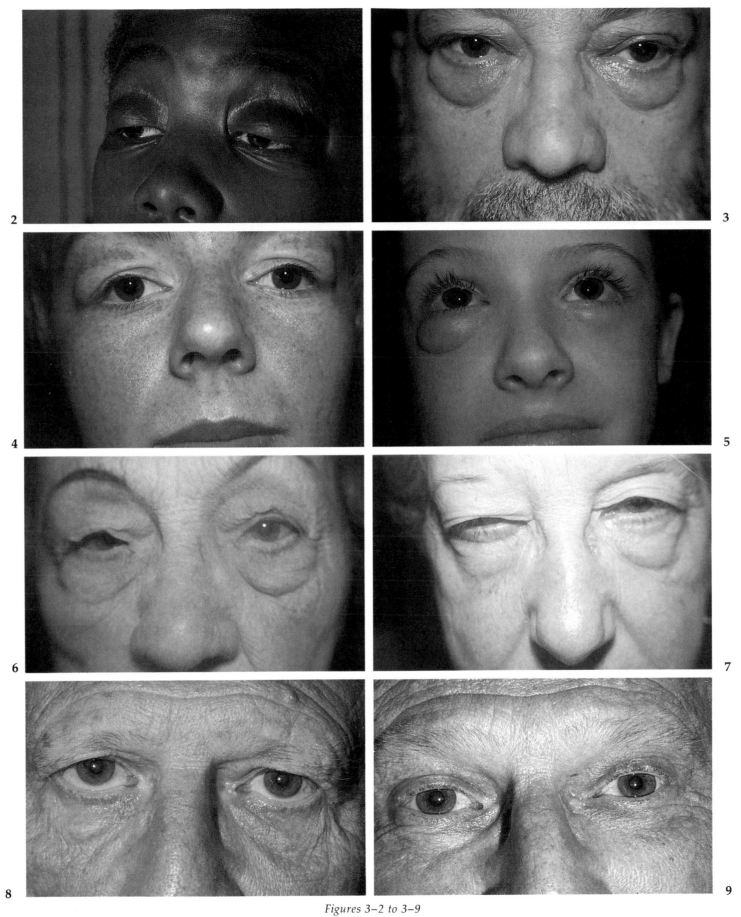

Figures 3–2 to 3–9

Figure 3–2   Upper lid blepharochalasis.
Figure 3–3   Blepharochalasis.
Figure 3–4   Blepharochalasis with congenital orbital septum defect.
Figure 3–5   Recurrent edema.

Figure 3–6   Dermachalasis.
Figure 3–7   Visual field constricted by severe dermachalasis.
Figure 3–8   Upright—skin hangs over lashes.
Figure 3–9   Patient in Fig. 3–8 when supine.

95

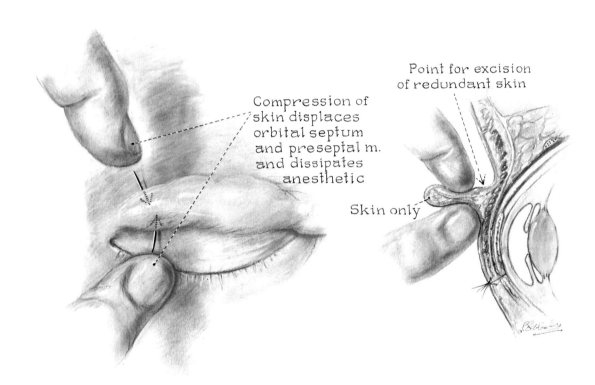

Compression of
skin displaces
orbital septum
and preseptal m.
and dissipates
anesthetic

Point for excision
of redundant skin

Skin only

Figure 3–11

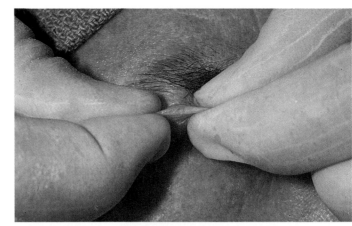

Figure 3–12 Pinch up redundant skin.
Figure 3–13 Skin will often stand in a ridge.
Figure 3–14 Blepharoplasty clamp. Eye closed.

12

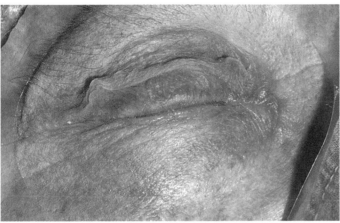

13

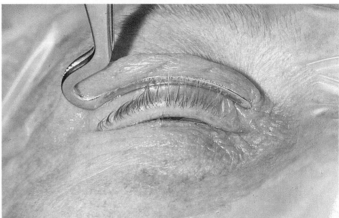

14

Figures 3–12 to 3–14

The excess skin of the upper lids is pinched between the thumb and forefinger (Figs. 3–11 and 3–12); when released, it will stand up as a small ridge across the lid (Fig. 3–13). A curved skin clamp (Storz No. E2507) is applied to this ridge, the lower blade at the level of the lid crease (Fig. 3–14), catching in its bite all the skin that can be pulled into the clamp with the lid *in the closed position* (Fig. 3–15). The clamp assures that the amount of skin removed will cause no postoperative difficulty with lid closure. The skin held in the clamp is excised by cutting along the proximal edge with curved scissors (Figs. 3–16 and 3–17). The scissors cut produces a slight crushing action that minimizes bleeding and produces a positive matching of the cut edges so that scar formation is minimized (Fig. 3–18). The skin edges, which are adherent after the scissors cut, are gently separated and as each cut vessel is exposed, it is occluded with mild cautery (Fig. 3–19). No undermining of the skin is necessary, but any slight irregularities are trimmed.

An 8–0 black silk suture is used to close the incision, beginning at the center so the alignment will be perfect (Fig. 3–24). Suturing then proceeds with closely placed interrupted stitches so that the skin is tightened evenly over the whole lid. At the nasal and temporal ends of the incision it is usually necessary to trim skin

Text continued on page 103

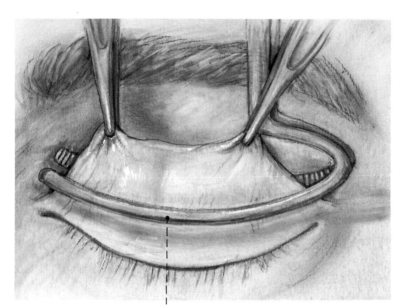

3–15

Clamp to be closed upon
base of skin pedicle

3–16

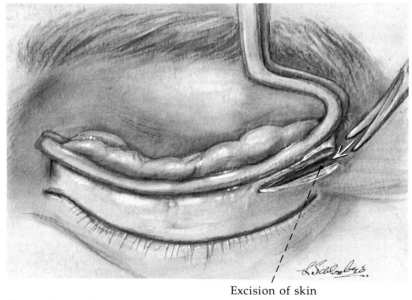

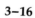

Excision of skin

Figures 3–15 and 3–16

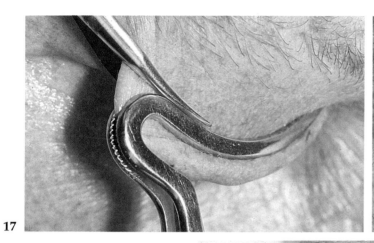
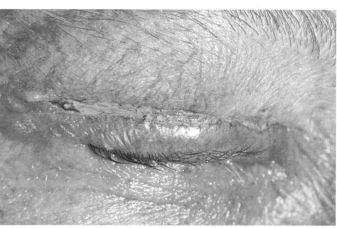
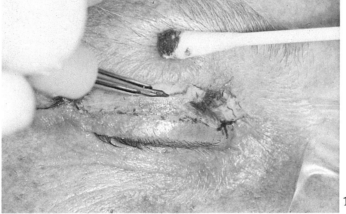

Figures 3–17 to 3–19

Figure 3–17   Cut under clamp.
Figure 3–18   Crush action of scissors gives temporary hemostasis.
Figure 3–19   Dry bleeders as they appear.

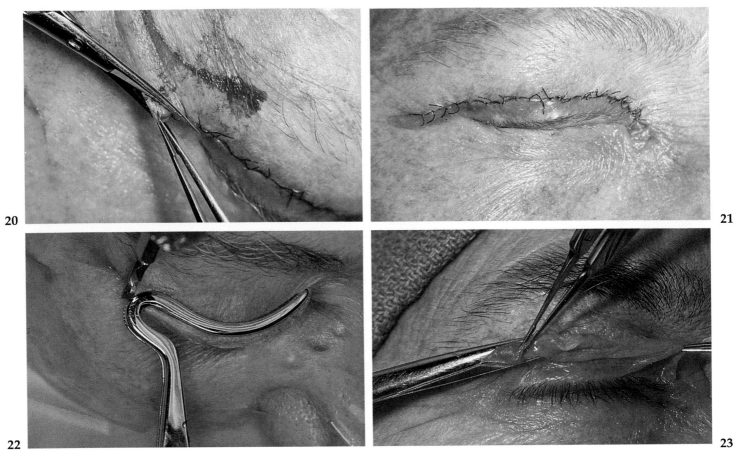

Figures 3–20 to 3–23

Figure 3–20 Excise "dog ears."
Figure 3–21 8–0 silk closure.
Figure 3–22 Scalpel can be used in place of scissors.
Figure 3–23 Skin can be excised after clamp removal.

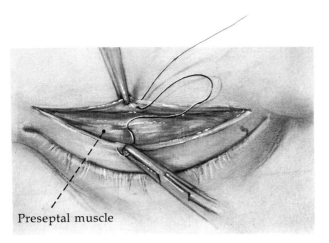

Preseptal muscle

Figure 3–24 Start suture in center.

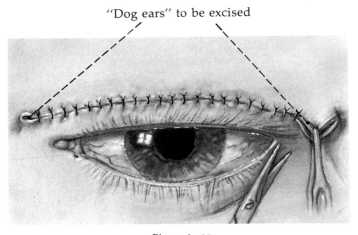

"Dog ears" to be excised

Figure 3–25

edges further to eliminate the puckers that are produced. This is done by grasping the pucker with forceps and excising the excess skin with scissors (Figs. 3–20, 3–25). The excision of the skin at the nasal end of the wound should not go below the canthal ligament. At the temporal end the excision is carried outward and is stopped just before the heavy skin of the temporal area is reached (Fig. 3–21). This avoids the webbing or hooding that would occur as the scar contracts if the incision were carried around the end of the canthi. Small natural wrinkles and crow's feet hide the fine linear scars that are produced by a properly placed incision. In older patients, in whom there may be heavy crow's feet and in whom the skin may occasionally be markedly redundant, it is possible to carry the excision farther temporally than in younger patients in whom the crow's feet are not as deeply furrowed and the postoperative scar would not be hidden.

The preseptal muscle, the orbital septum, and the levator aponeurosis should not be disturbed in doing a blepharoplasty for dermachalasis. It is hemorrhage into these tissues or trauma at the time of surgery that can cause a postoperative ptosis or a lid retraction.

VARIATIONS IN TECHNIQUE

It is much easier to cut the skin along the proximal edge of the blepharoplasty clamp with a knife (Fig. 3–22) than with scissors. However, the bleeding is much more profuse and difficult to control, as the advantage of the crushing action of the scissors is lost. The crushing action gives a short period of hemostasis so that each individual bleeder can be cauterized as the wound is gently opened.

On occasion, the blepharoplasty clamp is used merely to mark the amount of the skin that can be safely excised. This is done by placing the lower blade of the clamp along the premarked lid crease and catching in the clamp all the skin that can be picked up with the lid in the closed position. The upper edge of the incision is then lightly marked with a No. 15 scalpel blade. It is important that only the skin be marked and that the incision be made very lightly. The clamp is then carefully removed, and the skin that has been pinched in the clamp is pulled up in its initial ridge for excision with scissors (Fig. 3–23). For making this excision, we have found that the Storz scissors (No. 3668), which are slightly curved and lightweight but have a fairly heavy blade, give a clean cut. If the scissor blades are too light, the skin will tend to jam in the scissors and be folded as the blades are advanced across the lid. The assistant picks up the skin to be excised and elevates this as the cut is made. The surgeon, with another pair of forceps, keeps the folded excised skin away from the blades so that the planned excisional marks can be easily seen.

The excision of the ridge of skin gives matching edges that, when sutured, are so well mated that very little trimming is necessary except at the nasal and lateral ends of the excision.

103

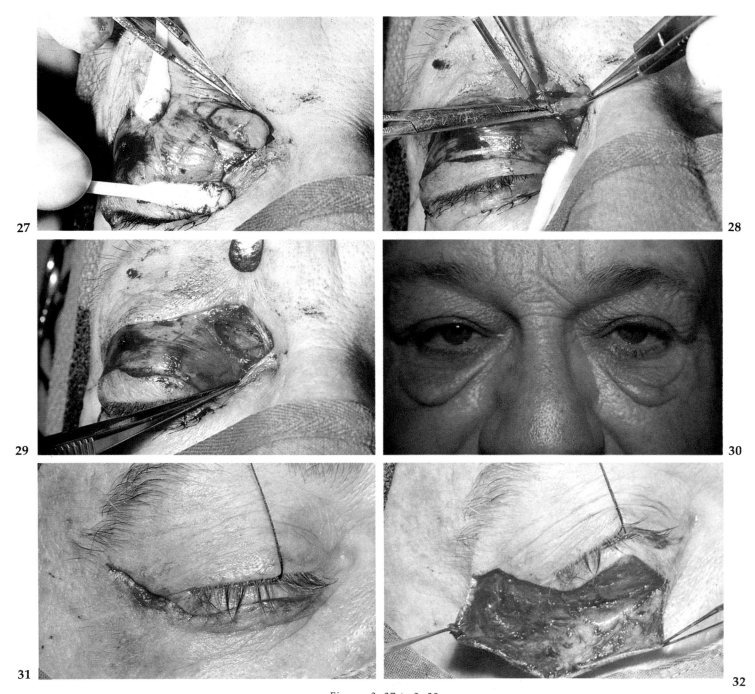

27

28

29

30

31

32

Figures 3–27 to 3–32

Figure 3–27 Apply pressure to prolapse orbital fat.
Figure 3–28 Excision of fat.
Figure 3–29 Inspection of base for bleeders.
Figure 3–30 Dermachalasis and skin edema.
Figure 3–31 Lower lid incision.
Figure 3–32 Dissect to level of orbital rim.

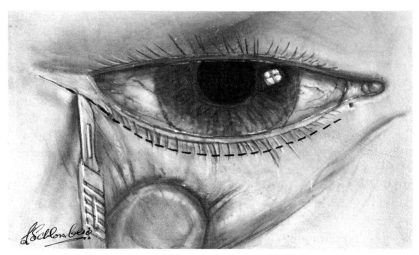

Figure 3–33

combined with the removal of only a small amount of skin just inferior to the lashes.

A skin incision is made 2 mm below the lash margin from 5 mm lateral to the punctum and carried out in a smooth curve to a point just temporal to the lateral canthus (Fig. 3–33). This incision is made just through the skin, with very light pressure exerted on the blade as it is passed across the proposed incisional line so that the skin is not distorted or rolled in front of the knife, which would produce an irregular cut. Sharp-pointed iris scissors are then used to complete the incision where the knife has not gone completely through the skin (Fig. 3–31). Dissection just beneath the skin and anterior to the level of the orbicularis muscle with the blunt-pointed Wescott scissors is carried as far down as the orbital rim (Figs. 3–32 and 3–34). It is often difficult to find a plane of cleavage anterior to the orbicularis, and moderate hemorrhage will be encountered. The dissection extends temporally as far as the lateral margin of the incision but not beyond. The edge of the

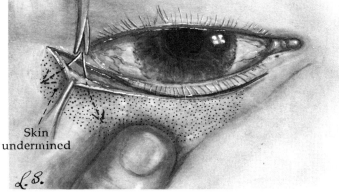

Skin
undermined

Figure 3–34

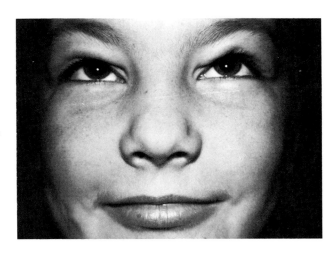

Figure 3–54

Preoperative—true blepharochalasis, with protrusion of orbital fat.

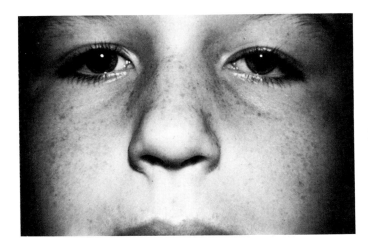

Figure 3–55

Postoperative—both fat and skin removed.

skin and muscle bleeding is important, and if fat is to be excised, extra care should be taken that a bleeder does not retract into the orbit. Use of mild pressure and eye pads of a nonadherent (Telfa) material without ointment for 24 hours reduces the chance of a delayed hemorrhage, as the patient keeps the lids quiet. However, if patients request that no bandage be employed, dark glasses are substituted. The patient is advised to keep the eyes closed as much as possible. Patients are discharged from the hospital in 24 hours without bandages, and as a rule, sutures that do not fall out are removed in four to five days. After 24 hours, a bland ointment is used over the incision for several weeks to keep the skin soft and prevent crusting.

Figures 3–50 and 3–51 are pre- and postoperative views of a patient with severe asthenopic symptoms preoperatively, relieved by the removal of the heavy skin of the upper lids.

Figures 3–52 and 3–53 are pre- and postoperative views of a woman who had skin and fat removed from both upper and lower lids.

Figures 3–54 and 3–55 show a true blepharochalasis in a young girl with protrusion of orbital fat. Fat and skin both were excised.

Ptosis of the Brow

Ptosis of the brow adds to the cosmetic and functional deformity of both dermachalasis and blepharochalasis. To correct it, relaxed skin and subcutaneous tissue of the forehead must be excised, producing a scar that is difficult to hide because of its location and the character of the skin. (The skin of the forehead resembles that of the cheek, with a thick dermis and subcutaneous tissue.) The lower incision line for the resection of the excess skin and supporting tissue must be as close to the brow hair line as possible, and the brow must be suspended during the immediate postoperative period by a deep absorbable suture so that no tension is placed on the skin closure. Bodian* suggests, in addition, a temporary supporting suture from the brow to be brought out through the skin above the upper edge of the incision and tied over silicone strips.

Cosmetics can aid in hiding the scar, but the only way to hide it completely is to do a brow and forehead lift, placing the incision above the hair line of the scalp.

Complications of Blepharoplasty

An all too frequently encountered postoperative complication is the patient's dissatisfaction with the results obtained, even though in the opinion of the surgeon the results are excellent. It behooves the surgeon to carefully screen patients for blepharoplasty. His role is to honestly try to improve the situation for the patient. To do

---

*Bodian, Martin: Paper delivered to meeting of Am. Soc. Ophthal. Plastic & Reconstructive Surgery, 1975.

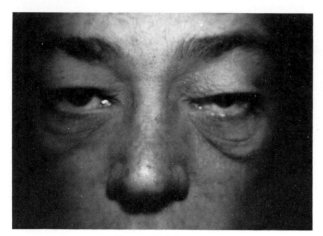

Figure 3–56

Preoperative.

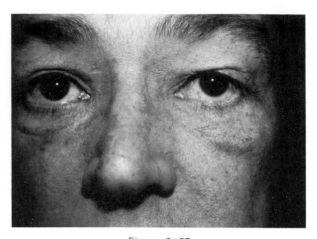

Figure 3–57

Postoperative residual fold — left upper lid — repaired with a secondary operation.

this he must understand what the patient really wishes to be accomplished, and more importantly, he must help the patient understand the limits of what can be done. If the patient is poorly enlightened by the surgeon and misconceptions and false expectations are not dispelled, the patient may be dissatisfied with even an excellent result. In addition, the surgeon must be able to recognize those patients whose psychological make-up precludes any possibility of their satisfaction regardless of what is done.

The tear status should be carefully evaluated in any patient being considered for blepharoplasty. If marginal tear production is detected or if the patient has any symptoms of dry eyes, blepharoplasty should be undertaken with the greatest caution. An asymptomatic eye with marginal tears may become symptomatic postoperatively as a result of a minimal widening of the palpebral fissure. Furthermore, a patient with no dry eye symptoms preoperatively may become symptomatic postoperatively as a result of his greater awareness of *any* sensation related to the eyes — even if the sensation was completely ignored prior to surgery.

Patient dissatisfaction when not enough skin is removed can easily be remedied as in the patient in Figures 3–56 and 3–57, in whom a second procedure was required on the left upper lid. The removal of too much skin from the upper lid does on occasion occur, but gravity and time help an overcorrection. However, when too much skin is removed from the lower lid an ectropion or lid retraction with scleral show is produced. The vertical drag of excessive skin excision is compounded by the effects of gravity on the relaxed lid tissues. For this reason, most operations on the lower lid are designed to tighten the skin by a lateral rather than a vertical shortening. When ectropion does occur (Fig. 3–58), skin from an upper lid is rotated as a flap to replace that which was excised (Fig. 3–59). If lid skin is not available, another donor site should be used, as discussed in Chapter 1 (Figs. 3–60 and 3–61).

A muscle imbalance after too vigorous removal of fat with a secondary hemorrhage has been seen. A sufficient waiting period should be allowed for resolution (six to eight months) before strabismus surgery is recommended.

Direct injury to the levator can cause ptosis; however, ptosis can occur following blepharoplasty in the absence of any direct injury to the levator just as it can occur following cataract or other intraocular operation. If postoperative ptosis occurs, it can be corrected by a small block resection (p. 61).

Carrying the incision in a curve around the inner or outer canthus can produce a wing-like scar as the scar contracts along its

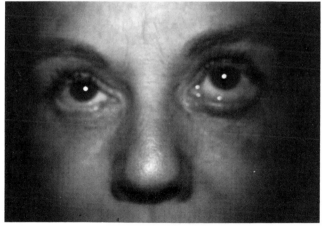

Figure 3–58

Blepharoplasty producing ectropion of the left lower lid, with corneal epithelial breakdown and blurring of vision.

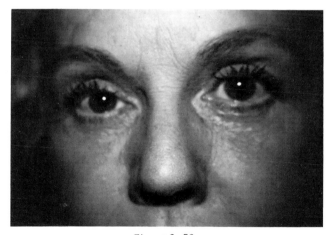

Figure 3–59

If available, skin from the upper lid can be used to repair lower lid ectropion as was done here.

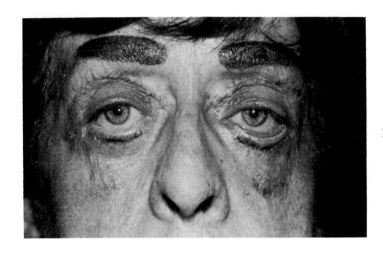

Figure 3–60

Ectropion following blepharoplasty.

Figure 3–61

Skin graft to left lower lid, seen 10 days postoperatively. Extensive burns in childhood made the postauricular, supraclavicular, and upper arm areas unsuitable as donor sites. A graft was taken from the inner thigh near the perineum.

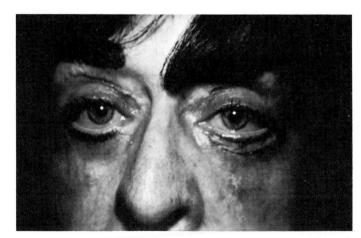

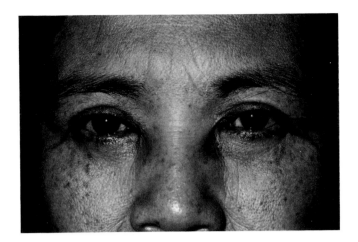

Figure 3–62

Patient referred with a wing-like scar as a result of a blepharoplasty incision carried around the medial canthus.

length (Fig. 3–62). A Z-plasty or skin graft is necessary for removal of these scars.

The lack of a good lid crease is an occasional complication of both blepharoplasty and ptosis surgery. To repair this defect and also to produce a lid crease in Orientals, an incision is made across the lid where the crease is desired. The skin edges are invaginated and fastened to the orbital septum and levator aponeurosis where they join at the upper edge of the tarsus (p. 84).

Deep orbital hemorrhages can occur and may cause increased orbital pressure, with possible occlusion of a central retinal vessel. This is an extremely rare occurrence, but it has been reported.

A check of the patient at three to four hours postoperatively for any undue discomfort or swelling should be done routinely. Should a retrobulbar hemorrhage occur, the wounds can be opened to release any trapped blood. However, this usually is an unsatisfactory procedure because the blood does not lie in a drainable pocket but instead infiltrates the tissues diffusely. Intraocular pressure and vision should be monitored and mannitol given if needed. If vision is threatened, an orbital decompression should be considered (see p. 159).

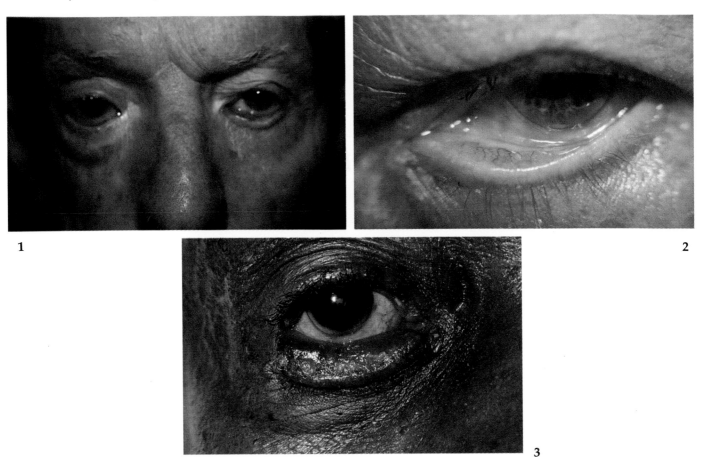

1   2

3

Figures 4–1 and 4–2 Senile ectropion.
Figure 4–3 Conjunctiva dries and becomes cornified.

An incision is made 1 mm below and parallel to the cilia line through skin and pretarsal muscle (Fig. 4–4, *A* and *B*). It is begun 4 mm lateral to the punctum, is carried to the lateral canthus, and then is extended about 1 cm outward in the crow's-foot crease. The skin and pretarsal and preseptal muscles (orbicularis) are separated from the tarsus and septum by undermining with blunt and sharp dissection to the level of the inferior cul-de-sac along the lid and to 1.5 cm below the lateral extension of the incision (Fig. 4–4C), but never below the junction of the thin skin of the lid and the heavier skin of the cheek. The size of this undermined pocket may seem quite large but it is needed to obtain the proper lateral and upward tension on the lid margin. Bleeding should be controlled by cautery to give a dry working field. This is often difficult, but extremely important because it reduces postoperative swelling and clot accumulation with undesirable secondary scarring.

At this stage of the procedure, the lid has been split into a posterior half, consisting of conjunctiva and tarsus with the intact lid margin containing the openings of the glands and a small band of skin containing the cilia, and an anterior half consisting of the orbicularis muscles and skin.

The posterior half of the lid is grasped at its margin with two Adson forceps about 2 cm apart. These forceps are brought together with a scissor-like motion to produce a vertical buckle. This gives an estimation of the amount of horizontal shortening (usually

Text continued on page 126

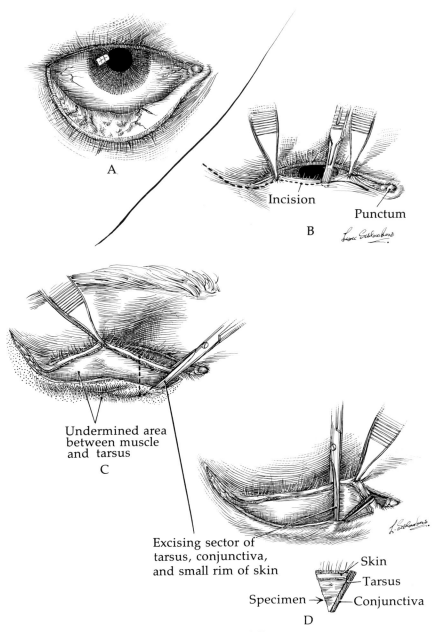

A

B

Incision

Punctum

C

Undermined area
between muscle
and tarsus

Excising sector of
tarsus, conjunctiva,
and small rim of skin

Skin

Tarsus

Specimen → Conjunctiva

D

Figure 4–4   Continued on following pages

1.0 to 1.5 cm) that will be necessary to tighten the lid margin and bring it in approximation with the globe. A triangle the width of this buckle is excised from the posterior portion of the lid. The base of the triangle is along the lid margin, and the apex is at the lower edge of the tarsus.

The lid is grasped just lateral to the midpoint by a firm bite of the Adson forceps and is put on stretch laterally. Canthotomy scissors are then used to cut the nasal side of the triangle, starting at the medial edge of the dissection and carrying down to the apex of the triangle just below the lower edge of tarsus. Marked arterial bleeding may be encountered from the superior and inferior arcuate vessels. On the nasal side of the incision the vessels are occluded with cautery. The temporal half of the lid is put on stretch by a medial pull of the Adson forceps, and the lateral side of the triangle is cut with scissors in a similar fashion to remove a wedge of tissue (Fig. 4–4D). To facilitate the control of bleeding, the cut edge of the tarsus can be grasped with the flat forceps (Storz No. 1901) with the blades paralleling the incision. This effectively stops all bleeding; then as the pressure on the blades is released, the cut vessels can be easily visualized and cauterized. The excised triangle consists of conjunctiva, tarsus, and the small rim of skin containing the cilia margin.

A 6–0 black silk suture is passed into the tarsus on the nasal portion of the lid, 2 mm from the incision and about 2 mm deep, to emerge in the incision (Fig. 4–4E). The needle is then passed into the temporal portion of the lid at this same depth and brought out through the tarsus 2 mm from the incision. Four loops are used in making this knot so that the lid margin is pulled together without buckling; the suture is left long. A lid plate is placed in the lower cul-de-sac; the 6–0 marginal suture is fastened to the knurled knob on the plate (Storz No. SP7-13456) to put the lid on stretch while the tarsus is closed with four to six interrupted 7–0 chromic catgut sutures (Fig. 4–4F). These are placed in the anterior edge of the tarsus and will be completely buried so that no suture material is exposed on the conjunctival surface. The 6–0 traction suture is then released from the lid plate and two 8–0 black silk sutures are placed, one posterior and one anterior to the initial suture, to give extra support to the lid margin and to produce a tight approximation of the wound edges in this critical area. These sutures are left long so they can ultimately be fastened to the skin of the lid. In this way, the ends are less likely to cause corneal irritation.

A base-up triangle is now removed from the skin and orbicularis muscle at the lateral end of the undermined area. The anterior half of the lid (skin and orbicularis muscle) is grasped in its midportion and mild tension exerted medially. One blade of the heavy scissors is inserted into the undermined area at the lateral edge and a vertical cut is made downward to the base of the undermined tissue. The free flap (skin and orbicularis muscle) is grasped with forceps and pulled laterally and upward over the vertical incision until it lies firmly against the posterior half of the lid. This overlap can then be excised precisely with scissors, and all bleeding points can be controlled (Fig. 4–4G).

The skin edges of the temporal vertical leg of the incision are undermined so that muscle-to-muscle suturing can be done, using two 5–0 double-armed chromic catgut sutures. The temporal undermining of the skin should be about 1 mm so that the knot of the muscle suture will lie slightly away from the skin suture line (Fig. 4–4H). A mattress stitch is used; thus, the base loop of the suture passes across the muscle fibers and is less likely to pull out. The first bite of the suture is made in the muscle on the free flap. A tie across the fibers of the muscle at this point helps to anchor the suture accurately. The two needles are then passed deep into the firm muscle temporally and brought out in the superficial pocket for a tie. Here again, using the mattress stitch places the knot across the muscle fibers and makes it less likely to pull out (Fig. 4–4H, detail). These sutures pull the orbicularis muscle temporally so that it acts as a sling to the lid, which is pulled upward and outward. This produces a slight overriding of the skin along the horizontal incision. The override is trimmed away and the skin of the horizontal and vertical incisions closed with 8–0 black silk suture placed at about 2 mm intervals (Fig. 4–4, I and J).

If at this stage of the procedure the roll of keratinized and thickened conjunctiva does not invert onto the tear layer, it must be excised. This roll of conjunctiva is picked up with Adson forceps and excised with scissors and cautery to remove the subconjunctival build-up of inflammatory tissue. No suturing is usually necessary to close, as the denuded area will rapidly epithelialize.

The long ends of the three sutures in lid margin (the 6–0 in the mid-tarsus and the 8–0 sutures posterior and anterior to it) are brought forward over the lid margin and fastened to the skin by a single 8–0 black silk suture. In this way, they will not rub on the cornea.

The eye is dressed with a nonadherent pad and mild pressure dressing for 24 hours and then is left uncovered. The silk sutures are left in for a week: during this time a small amount of ointment is put along the skin incision each evening (Figs. 4–5 and 4–6).

Noncicatricial Ectropion of the Upper Lid

Noncicatricial ectropion of the upper lid, in our experience, does not occur in adults because gravity tends to make even a relaxed lid hug the globe. It can occur as a congenital anomaly as a result of an overlong horizontal dimension of the lid and a relaxed orbicularis muscle (Fig. 4–7). The congenital upper lid ectropion can be cured by a full thickness block resection of the lid (Fig. 4–8), which shortens it horizontally and tightens the tarsal and preseptal portion of the orbicularis muscle (Fig. 4–9).

Operation for Correction of Ectropion of the Lower Punctum

We have successfully used Byron Smith's lazy "T" procedure* for the correction of ectropion of the lower punctum. The vertical

*Smith, B.: The "lazy-T" correction of ectropion of the lower punctum. Arch. Ophthalmol. 94:1149, 1976.

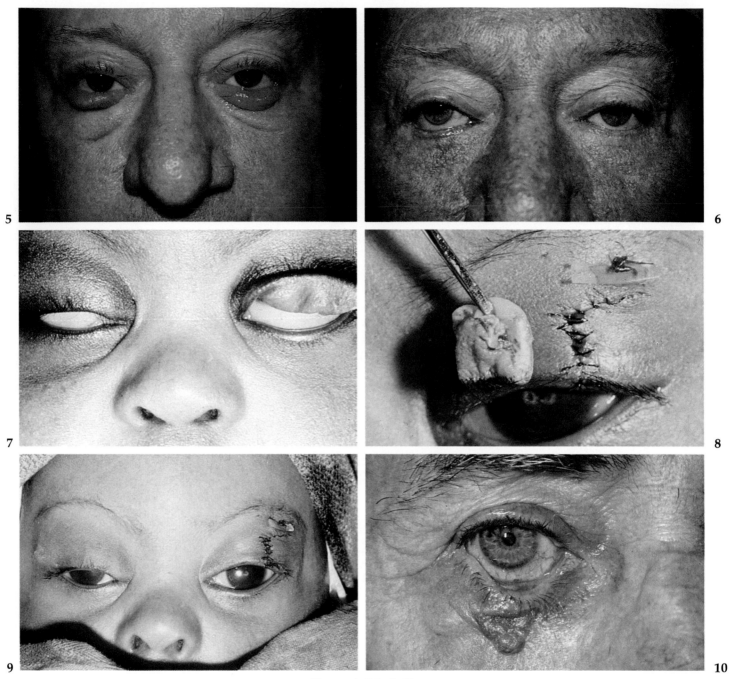

5

6

7

8

9

10

Figures 4–5 to 4–10

Figure 4–5   Preoperative ectropion.
Figure 4–6   Postoperative.
Figure 4–7   Congenital upper lid ectropion.
Figures 4–8 and 4–9   Full thickness lid resection repaired the deformity.
Figure 4–10   Recurrent basal cell carcinoma which had received four previous operations plus radiation therapy. Both the thin skin of the lid and the heavy skin of the cheek are invaded by tumor.

dimension of the conjunctiva and tarsus is shortened by the excision of 5 to 6 mm of tissue, and the relaxed lid is horizontally tightened by the resection of a full thickness base-up triangle of lid.

A lacrimal probe in the canaliculus outlines the tract. The lid is everted by grasping it with Adson forceps at its midpoint. A 1 cm horizontal incision 3 mm below the canaliculus is made with a

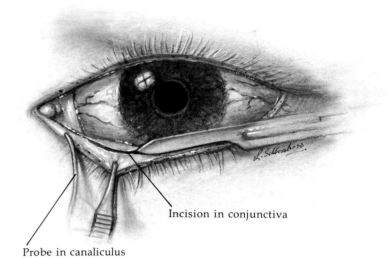

Figure 4–11

Incision in conjunctiva

Probe in canaliculus

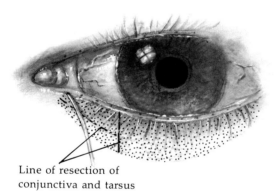

Line of resection of
conjunctiva and tarsus

Figure 4–12

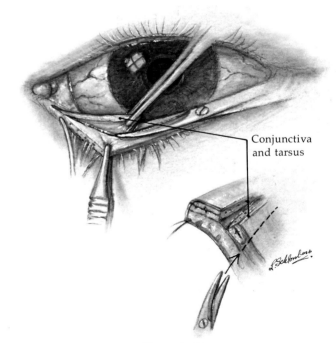

Conjunctiva
and tarsus

Figure 4–13

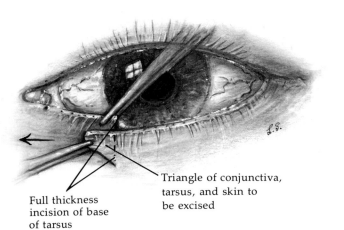

Figure 4–14

Full thickness
incision of base
of tarsus

Triangle of conjunctiva,
tarsus, and skin to
be excised

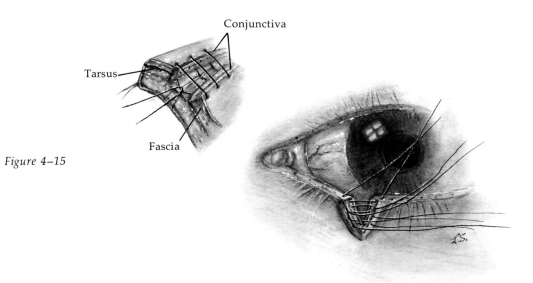

Conjunctiva

Tarsus

Fascia

Figure 4–15

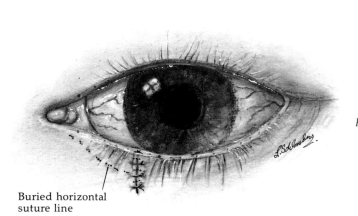

Figure 4–16

Buried horizontal
suture line

No. 15 blade through conjunctiva and tarsus (Fig. 4–11). The inferior margin of the incision is undermined for 5 mm and this area resected (Figs. 4–12 and 4–13).

A vertical full thickness incision of the lid is made with scissors to the base of the tarsus 3 mm temporal to the punctum. The temporal half of the lid is pulled nasally to overlap the vertical cut to estimate the amount of shortening required, and a base-up triangle of this amount is excised (Fig. 4–14).

The horizontal incision is closed with interrupted 7–0 absorbable sutures with the knots buried (Fig. 4–15). The vertical full thickness lid incision is closed in two layers as has been described (Fig. 4–16).

Cicatricial Ectropion

Cicatricial ectropion occurs when the tissues of the lid are invaded by tumor or involved in secondary scarring from healing after trauma or infection. A basal cell carcinoma—with its components of ulceration, invasion, and cicatrization—is the chief offender among the tumors (Fig. 4–10). Iatrogenically produced scarring from surgery or irradiation may play a part in this problem. Scarring following trauma, burns, or bacterial or viral infections produces such varied pictures that only basic surgical techniques can be presented here to aid in the treatment.

The correction of a cicatricial ectropion consists of removing the abnormal scarred tissue and replacing it with a substitute, either from the adjoining area or from some other part of the body. We have stressed the remarkable softness of the lid skin and its lack of subcutaneous fat and fibrous tissue. It is of utmost importance to replace the damaged tissue with like material. The best source is other lid tissue from either the same or the opposite eye. If this is not available, the next most pliable skin in the male is foreskin. There is a color difference that later has to be corrected with Covermark or a similar matching cosmetic, but the texture match is excellent. If the patient is female (or if foreskin is not available in the male), skin from behind the ear will give a good texture and color match and, if available, is generally the donor skin of choice. Other donor sites are the supraclavicular area, the medial aspect of the upper arm near the axilla, or the inner portion of the thigh close to the perineum if the skin is relatively free from hair. Skin of the forehead, cheek, or temporal area is definitely of a different character and gives a poor cosmetic and functional result. Figure 4–17 shows a case of severe scarring and corneal ulceration following herpes zoster in which a large skin graft was required to reconstruct the upper lid.

The skin graft should be separated from subcutaneous tissue and made as thin as possible. It is placed epithelium side down on a wood board and stretched and pinned to the board with 25-gauge hypodermic needles (Fig. 4–18). These needles are better than pins, as the plastic end makes a good handle for directing the point of the needle. The subcutaneous material is removed with curved Wescott scissors, cutting with the curve of the scissors rather than with the points. In this way, the loose subcutaneous material can be cut

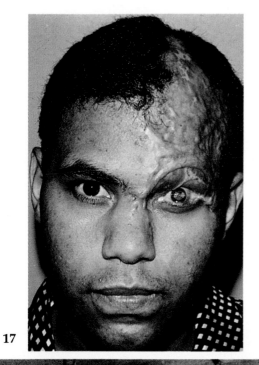

Figure 4–17 Severe scarring following herpes zoster infection– corneal decompensation due to exposure.
Figure 4–18 Foreskin pinned to a board for removal of subcutaneous tissue.
Figure 4–19 Conjunctiva and tarsus are dissected free from scar.
Figure 4–20 Graft carefully sutured in place.
Figure 4–21 Six months postoperatively; a brow had been grafted in addition.

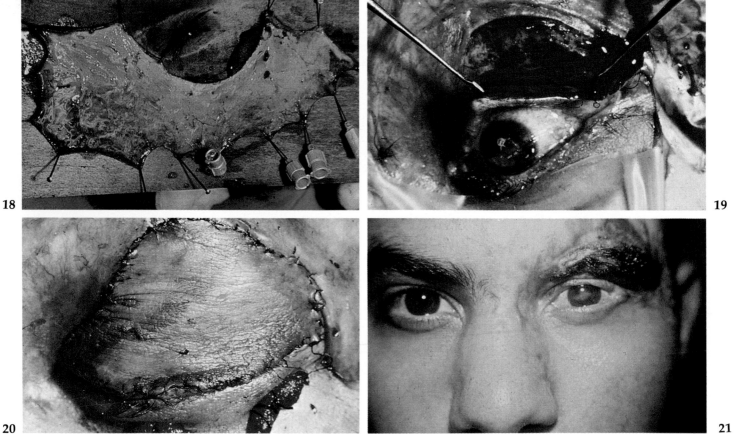

Figures 4–17 to 4–21

away with less likelihood of buttonholing the graft. Actually, an occasional small hole in the graft does no harm, for it permits the draining of trapped fluid. However, it is better to position the drainage holes deliberately rather than to inadvertently cut them while preparing the graft.

The bed for the graft must be free of all contracted scarred bands that would cause a continuation of lid retraction (Fig. 4–19). Much of the preseptal and pretarsal (orbicularis) muscle can be removed without producing any problem with lid closure. The graft itself is sutured in place with interrupted 8–0 black silk sutures, making sure the edge-to-edge apposition is perfect (Fig. 4–20). A mild pressure bandage over a nonadherent gauze dressing without ointment is applied for 48 hours. Thereafter, the graft should be covered with a bland ointment so that it does not dry out. Ointment is not used in the primary dressing, as it tends to get into the wound and delay good edge-to-edge union (Fig. 4–21).

It is difficult to make a lower lid stay up in place unless it has a supporting tissue such as the tarsus. Therefore, if the tarsus has been involved in the scar and must be removed for relaxation of the lid margin, it must be replaced by similar tissue such as tarsus from the other lid or preserved sclera. If the skin has also been involved in the scar, a flap of skin rotated from the upper lid will be required rather than a free graft, because it is not practical to overlay a free tarsal or scleral graft with a free skin graft.

The primary goal is to restore lid function and to improve the appearance of the orbital area. Each case presents an individual problem and must be handled using the basic principles discussed in Chapter 1.

ENTROPION

Senile and Spastic Entropion

Senile entropion of the lower lid is caused by a combination of laxness of tissues and irritative factors. Although pure atonic entropion can occur, irritation is often present as is the case with conjunctivitis, corneal abrasion from inturned lashes, or inflammation following intraocular surgery. The irritation may lead to a spastic component. Entropion procedures can be categorized as (1) resections or transpositions of pieces of skin or tarsus, (2) cautery, (3) selected orbicularis lapping or tightening procedures, and (4) lid suturing procedures.

The anatomy of the lower lid is shown in Figure 4–22. In cross section are shown the skin, superficial fascia, and orbicularis, which can be divided into the pretarsal muscle and the preseptal portion which lies just anterior to the orbital septum. Posterior to this are the capsulopalpebral fascia (analogous to the levator aponeurosis in the upper lid), which joins the sheath of the inferior oblique muscle, and the expansion of Tenon's fascia from the insertion of the inferior rectus muscle. The capsulopalpebral fascia attaches with the orbital septum to the tarsus at its anterior inferior edge. The inferior palpebral muscle, which is analogous to Mueller's muscle in the upper lid, also originates in the fascial

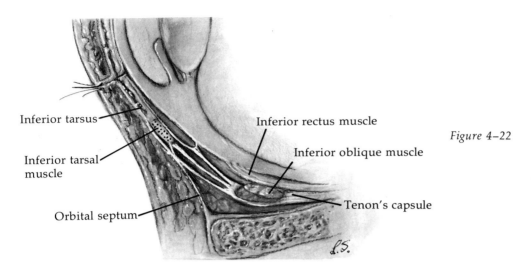

Inferior tarsus

Inferior tarsal muscle

Orbital septum

Inferior rectus muscle

Inferior oblique muscle

Tenon's capsule

Figure 4–22

sheaths of the inferior oblique and inferior rectus muscles and inserts to the posterior inferior tarsal edge. A strand of fascia attaches to the conjunctiva in the fornix which is the analog to the superior forniceal suspensory ligament.

In senile entropion, many or all of the following changes can be found. Some degree of enophthalmos occurs due to absorption of orbital fat. This reduces the pressure of the globe against the tarsi. The skin and superficial fascia become atonic, redundant, and less adherent to the orbicularis in the preseptal area. The lower preseptal muscle becomes less fixed to the underlying orbital septum, reducing its pressure on the base of the tarsus. Finally, the lower lid retractors (capsulopalpebral fascia and inferior palpebral muscle) become relaxed and atonic. All of these changes tend to decrease the support to the lower tarsus, allowing its base to rotate anterior-

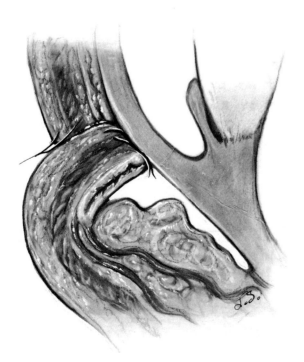

Figure 4–23
Lower lid entropion.

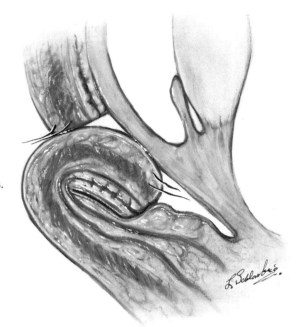

Figure 4–24

Severe entropion may have complete inversion of the tarsus.

ly, resulting in its inward tumbling of 90 degrees (Fig. 4–23) or even up to 180 degrees (Fig. 4–24). The typical clinical appearance is shown in Figure 4–25. If there is ocular irritation, spasm of the pretarsal orbicularis and upriding of the preseptal orbicularis exacerbate the problem. The muscle of Riolan, implicated by some observers, is so small that it is doubtful whether it contributes much to the problem.

Correction of entropion by strategically placed sutures dates back to Hippocrates; the procedure has been modified by Gaillard, Arlt, Snellen, Stellwag, and more recently, Feldstein and Quickert.* The high success rate and ease of performance of this operation make it an ideal procedure. We have had very good results with the following procedure in the treatment of senile and spastic entropion, and we feel it is superior to those described by some of the above authors. The high incidence of success depends on closely observing small points in the technique.

OPERATION FOR CORRECTION OF SPASTIC
ENTROPION

The lid is anesthetized with a subcutaneous and subconjunctival injection of 1 per cent lidocaine (Fig. 4–26). It is then everted,

---

*Beard, C. H.: *Ophthalmic Surgery*, Blakiston Co., Philadelphia, 1914 (Hippocrates reference); Gaillard, A. L.: *Suture pour l'entropion. Ann Ocul* 18:241, 1847; Arlt, C. F.: *Die Krankheiten des Auges fur praktische Aertze geschildert.* A. Credner, Prague, Vol. 3, 1854; Snellen, H.: Suture for entropion. *Cong. Internat. d'opht.* (Paris) 1863; Stellwag von, C.: *Ein neues Verfahren gegen einwartsgekehrte Wimptern. Allgem Wien Med Ztg* 28:527, 1883; Feldstein, M.: Correction of senile entropion. Ophthalmol. Surg. 1:20, 1970; Quickert, M. H., and Rathbun, E.: Suture repair of entropion. Arch. Ophthalmol. 85:304, 1971.

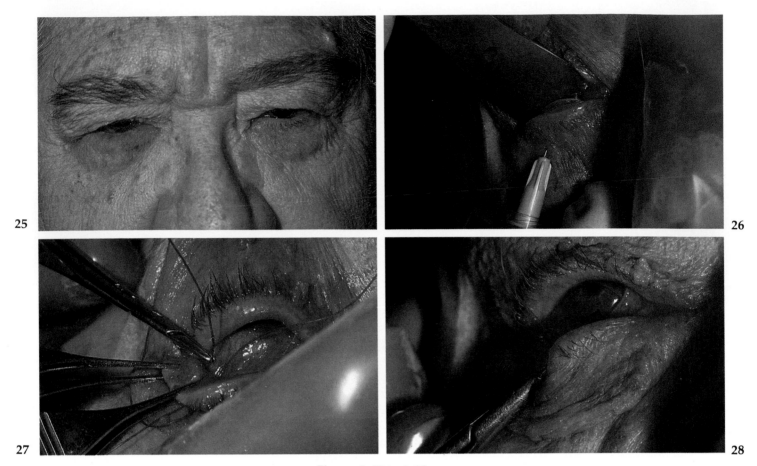

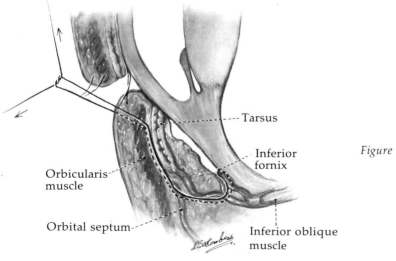

Figures 4–25 to 4–28

Figure 4–25 Right lower lid entropion.
Figure 4–26 Local anesthesia.
Figure 4–27 Suture is passed deep in the cul de sac.
Figure 4–28 Suture is brought out just inferior to the lash line.

Tarsus

Inferior fornix

Orbicularis muscle

Orbital septum

Inferior oblique muscle

Figure 4–29

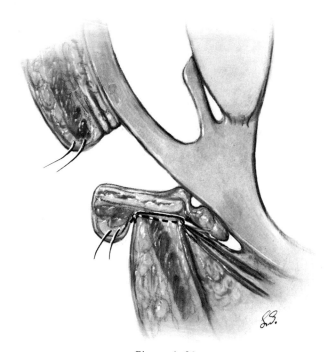

Figure 4–30

Initial overcorrection is desired.

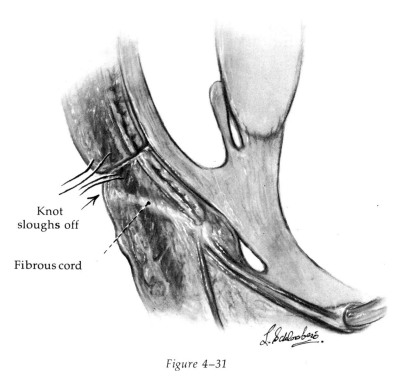

Knot
sloughs off

Fibrous cord

Figure 4–31

Desired effect of the sutures.

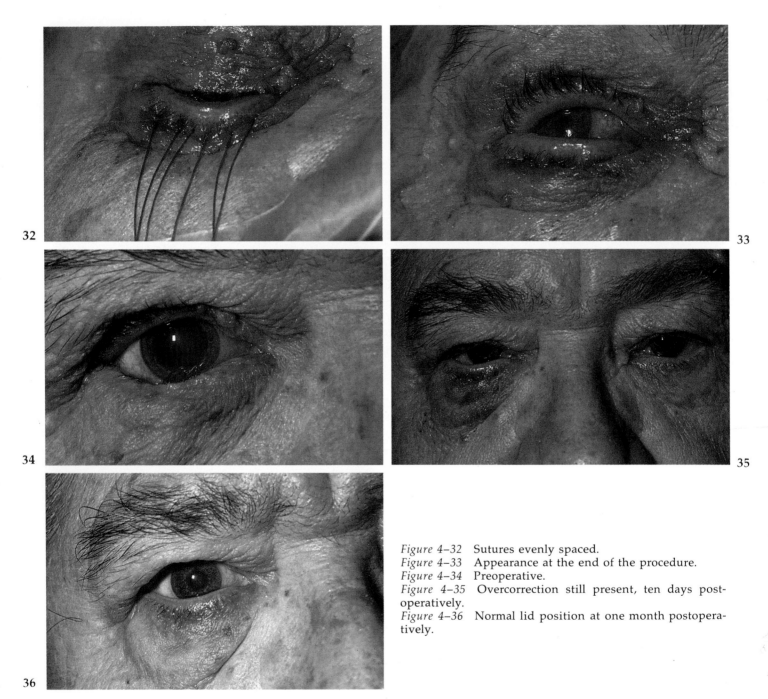

Figure 4–32 Sutures evenly spaced.
Figure 4–33 Appearance at the end of the procedure.
Figure 4–34 Preoperative.
Figure 4–35 Overcorrection still present, ten days postoperatively.
Figure 4–36 Normal lid position at one month postoperatively.

Figures 4–32 to 4–36

and one needle of a double-armed suture of 4–0 chromic catgut (Ethicon No. 751-G) — angled so the suaged end does not hit the globe — is passed deep in the cul-de-sac, through the conjunctiva, to engage the inferior orbital fascial and muscular tarsal attachments (Fig 4–27). The needle is then passed just anterior to the tarsus, to exit through the skin 1 to 2 mm inferior to the lash line (Fig. 4–28). Figure 4–29 demonstrates the desired position of the sutures.

The second arm of the suture is passed in a similar fashion 2 to 3 mm laterally. Two additional sutures are then placed at equal distances along the lid (Fig. 4–32). The sutures are tied, causing eversion of the lid to the point that the tarsus is *rotated outward 30 to 45 degrees from the vertical position* (Fig. 4–33). In this way, the inferior fascial and muscular attachments to the tarsus are gathered (Fig. 4–30), and ultimately a band of fibrous tissue replaces the suture to secure the shortened fascia to the tarsus orbicularis and skin as shown (Fig. 4–31). The knots slough off in 14 to 21 days.

Figure 4–34 shows the preoperative appearance. At ten days, mild overcorrection is present (Fig. 4–35); but at one month postoperatively, the lid is in normal position (Fig. 4–36). We feel that this initial overcorrection is essential to the success of the procedure. If there is not an initial overcorrection, the fibrous bands produced by the reaction to the catgut suture stretch and may permit a return of the entropion. In rare instances, an excessive immediate overcorrection is obtained. If this persists for more than two weeks postoperatively, the knots can be cut off at skin level to permit the sutures to retract, eliminating the overcorrection.

In a small percentage of cases entropion recurs. The same three-stitch procedure can be repeated.

Because this procedure is simple and highly successful and can be done on an outpatient basis, it has replaced other, more complicated methods.

Cicatricial Entropion and Trichiasis

Spastic entropion of the upper lid is rare because the large tarsal plate and the well-developed retractors prevent the inturning of the lid margin. On the other hand, cicatricial entropion with the associated trichiasis is relatively common. Trachoma, recurrent infection of the glands of the lid, tumor, and trauma distort the tarsus as healing occurs. Scarring produces an inward curving of the tarsal plate that brings the lashes into contact with the cornea (Fig. 4–37). Ocular discomfort causes the patient to constantly pull the lid away from the globe, breaking off lashes which then become short stubs even more devastating to the cornea. The process is a self-perpetuating and worsening condition. Corneal ulcers, producing corneal scars, reduce visual acuity and in severe cases can cause blindness.

If the trichiasis consists of a few large cilia, they can be removed by electrolysis. Very fine lashes can be removed by repeated freezing and thawing of the lash margin to −20 °C as measured by a

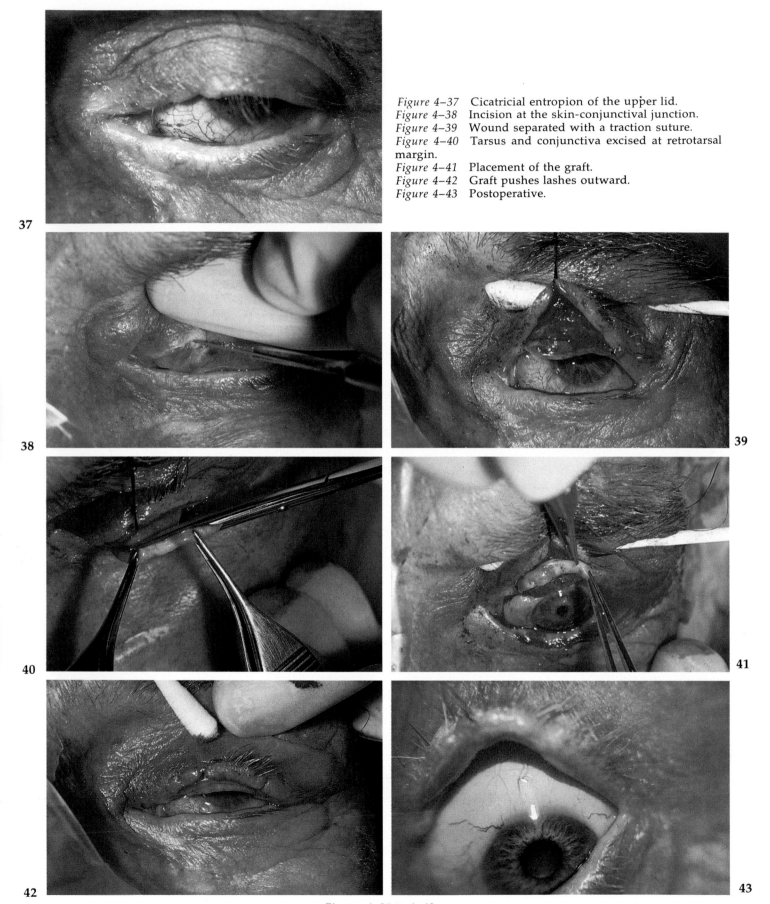

Figure 4–37 Cicatricial entropion of the upper lid.
Figure 4–38 Incision at the skin-conjunctival junction.
Figure 4–39 Wound separated with a traction suture.
Figure 4–40 Tarsus and conjunctiva excised at retrotarsal margin.
Figure 4–41 Placement of the graft.
Figure 4–42 Graft pushes lashes outward.
Figure 4–43 Postoperative.

Figures 4–38 to 4–43

thermocouple, using a retinal-detachment-type cryoprobe. The freeze-thaw cycle may be repeated two or three times. It produces little reaction and is accepted well by patients. However, since depigmentation of the lid margin occasionally occurs, cryoepilation should not be used in Negroes.

For trichiasis of a greater degree, a variety of tarsal fracturing and rotating procedures have been used. However, we have found that a tarsal conjunctival graft at the posterior edge of the lid gives the most satisfactory results. A strip of tarsus and conjunctiva is transplanted from the retrotarsal edge from either the same or the other upper lid to create a new, smooth inner lid margin. The graft is placed in a bed of tarsus just behind the row of offending lashes. Here it forms a new inner lid margin and actually pushes the lashes outward, away from the cornea.

OPERATION FOR CORRECTION OF MODERATE
ENTROPION AND TRICHIASIS OF THE UPPER
LID — TARSOCONJUNCTIVAL GRAFT TO LID
MARGIN

Local anesthesia of 1 per cent lidocaine (Xylocaine) is injected with a 30-gauge needle beneath the skin across the width of the lid, 5 mm superior to the lash line. The needle is withdrawn to the puncture point just beneath the skin, the lid everted, and the needle passed into the deep tissues of the upper fornix—injecting lidocaine to balloon out the conjunctiva.

A 4–0 black silk suture through the anterior lid margin gives traction as the lid is everted on a Desmarres retractor. With the lid margin firmly fixed, an incision behind the most posterior lashes can be made across the full width of the tarsus to the depth of 3 mm. This incision line usually falls at about the posterior edge of the lid margin considerably behind the gray line (Fig. 4–38). The traction suture will be in the anterior half of the lid and will produce a gaping of the wound (Fig. 4–39).

The lid is grasped firmly in its everted position by two Adson forceps at the nasal and temporal sides of the retrotarsal margin. A 2 mm strip of tarsus with attached conjunctiva is excised across the whole width of the lid (Fig. 4–40). This is best done with straight canthotomy scissors since the tarsus is firm and the cut should be exact. Reattachment of the conjunctiva and Mueller's muscle to the upper edge of the tarsus can be done with 7–0 chromic catgut in a running stitch. However, in many instances we have not closed this wound and no untoward results have been noted.

The tarsal graft, with a conjunctival covering on one side, is now placed in the lid margin incision (Fig. 4–41). The posterior edge is sutured first, using buried 7–0 chromic catgut sutures; care must be taken that no knot is exposed that might rub on the cornea. The anterior edge is then sutured in a similar manner. At the end of the procedure, the tarsal graft has become the posterior lid margin, pushing the anterior half of the lid outward 2 mm (Fig. 4–42). No ointment is placed in the eye for 24 hours. After 24 hours, a steroid ointment may be used morning and night and an

141

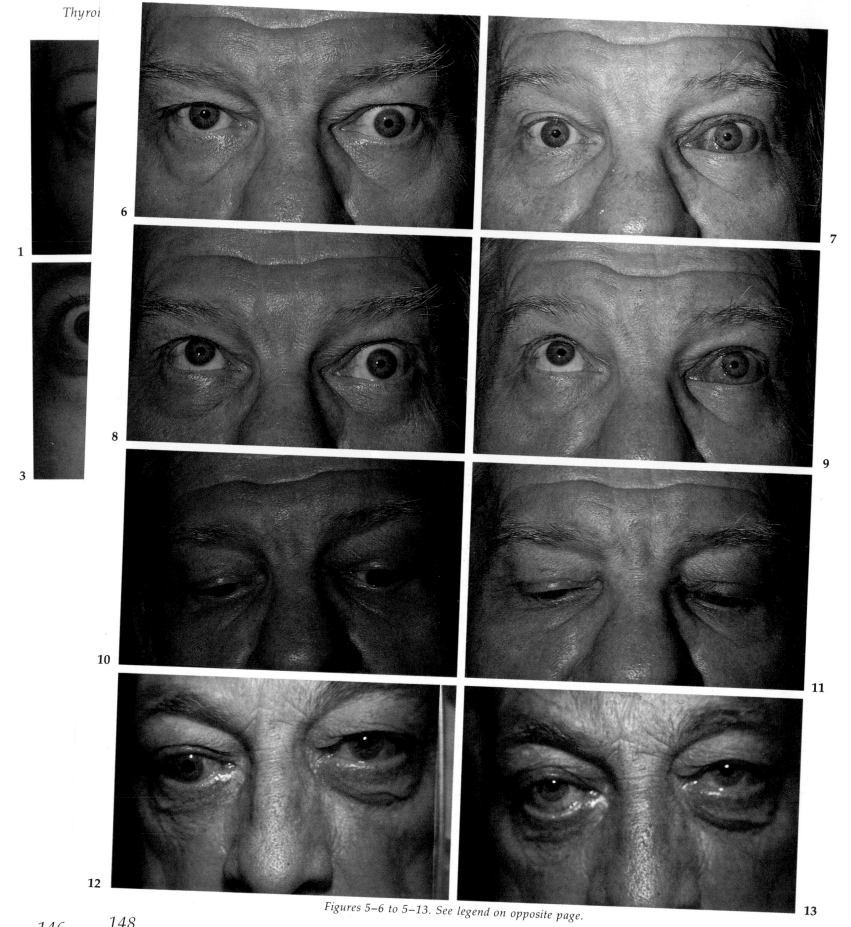

Figures 5–6 to 5–13. See legend on opposite page.

1

3

6

7

8

9

10

11

12

13

OPERATION TO RECESS THE INFERIOR
RECTUS MUSCLE

A recession of the inferior rectus muscle should be done under general anesthesia, as injections around the muscle or a retrobulbar injection further distorts the already tight inferior orbit.

Using forced duction, the eye is rotated upward to check the amount of retraction. If it can be elevated to the horizontal, a recession of 4 to 6 mm is indicated; if it cannot be elevated to the horizontal, the recession will of necessity be greater and may place the insertion behind the equator. If the orbit is fixed and the eye cannot be rotated upward at all, a tenotomy of the muscle should be done.

With the lid speculum in place, two double-armed, 6–0 black silk traction sutures are placed in the episclera at the limbus at nine and three o'clock.

The eye is rotated up as much as possible with the two traction sutures, which are then fixed to the knurled knob of the speculum. An incision through the conjunctiva is made directly over the insertion of the inferior rectus muscle. Bleeding is carefully controlled by cautery. The muscle is picked up with hooks and freed from the overlying conjunctiva and check ligaments. A 5–0 absorbable suture is placed in the muscle at the insertion, using a mattress stitch tied and double-locked. The muscle is then cut from its insertion on the globe, and the bleeders of the stump and globe are cauterized. With the muscle free from the globe, further dissection of the check ligaments can be done.

The fascial bands between the inferior rectus and the lower lid must be severed. A 4–0 black silk suture is placed in the skin of the lower lid for traction, and the lid is everted over a Desmarres retractor. The fascial bands between the inferior rectus muscle and the inferior edge of the tarsus are put on stretch and cut across the whole width of the lid, the incision being carried almost to the skin. In a very tight orbit, it is difficult to cut all the retractors.

In severe cases, the eye has to be held in an elevated position during the initial healing period. The needles of the two traction sutures at nine and three o'clock on the globe are passed into the fornix of the upper lid and brought out through the skin, where they are tied over small cotton pledgets. Enough tension is put on these sutures to rotate the globe to 30 degrees above the horizontal. The conjunctival incision over the insertion of the inferior rectus muscle is not closed. The ends of the 4–0 black silk traction suture in the lower lid are pulled upward and fastened to adhesive tape on the brow so that the lower lid is put on stretch to prevent the cut retractors from immediately rejoining. This is a true Frost suture (p. 58).

Figures 5–6 to 5–13

Figures 5–6, 5–8, 5–10 Tight left inferior rectus and upper lid retraction.
Figures 5–7, 5–9, 5–11 Postoperative recession of left inferior rectus (and cutting of retractors of the lower lid). Upper lid retraction disappears.
Figures 5–12 and 5–13 Preoperative and postoperative recession of the right inferior rectus without cutting the lower lid retractors. Postoperative lower lid retraction.

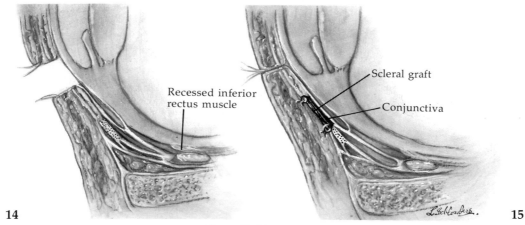

14

15

Figure 5–14

Retractors of the lower lid attach to the inferior tarsal border.

Figure 5–15

A scleral implant is placed between the retractors and the tarsus.

Decadron is injected beneath the skin at the level of the preseptal muscle across the lower lid, and the eye is dressed with steroid ointment and an eye pad. The eye is redressed in 24 hours, but the traction sutures to the globe and lid are left in place for four days.

OPERATION TO CORRECT RETRACTION OF LOWER LID

If all the retractors of the lower lid have not been cut during the primary operation on the inferior rectus muscle, there is retraction of the lid causing marked scleral show in the primary position and on downward gaze, and a second operative procedure is necessary (Figs. 5–12 and 5–13). At this stage, cutting the retractors of the lower lid is not sufficient and a scleral implant must be placed between the inferior border of the tarsus and the retractors of the lid (Figs. 5–14 and 5–15).

A horizontal incision is made in the skin of the lid starting 4 mm below the punctum and extending laterally parallel to the lid margin to a point 3 mm in from the lateral canthus (Fig. 5–16). First, a light, smooth, slightly curved incision is made with a No. 15 Bard-Parker blade. This outline is completely opened with sharp-pointed iris scissors, and the skin is undermined upward as far as the cilia and downward for 1 cm. Rake retractors give exposure as the dissection is carried through the preseptal muscle and fascia to the lower edge of the tarsus. The retractors of the lower lid are cut at the inferior border of the tarsus. A lid plate or muscle hook that is placed in the lower cul-de-sac can be seen to shine through the conjunctiva and can act as a guide to the completeness of the dissection (Fig. 5–17). A piece of preserved sclera is then cut in a roughly rectangular shape, with the corners rounded. The rectangle is 2 cm wide; the vertical dimension is three times the amount of retraction to be corrected. The scleral insert is sutured to the lower edge of the tarsus (Fig. 5–18) and to the retractors of the lower lid (Fig. 5–19) with interrupted stitches of 7–0 chromic catgut.

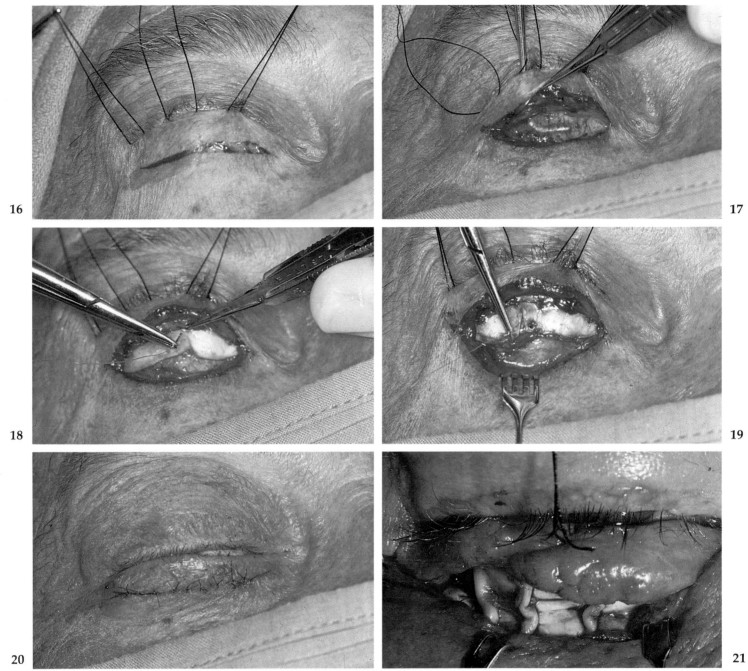

Figures 5–16 to 5–21

Figures 5–16 and 5–17 Incision is carried down to conjunctiva.
Figures 5–18 and 5–19 Donor sclera is sutured in place.
Figure 5–20 Skin closure.
Figure 5–21 Corrugations can be used for vertical stiffness.

The preseptal muscles are permitted to fall into place, and the skin is closed with interrupted stitches of 8–0 black silk (Fig. 5–20). A fairly tight pressure dressing is put in place for 48 hours; the skin sutures are removed in six days. Although others have advocated placing the implant from the conjunctival surface, we have found the skin approach more satisfactory, as the conjunctiva stretches easily to cover the graft and there is no suture line to rub on the globe.

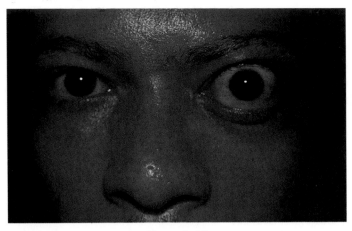

Figure 5–38

Unilateral thyroid exophthalmos.

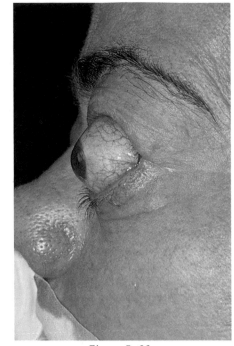

Figure 5–39

Lids may retract behind the globe.

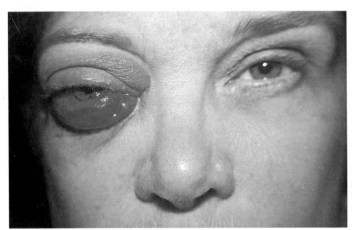

Figure 5–40

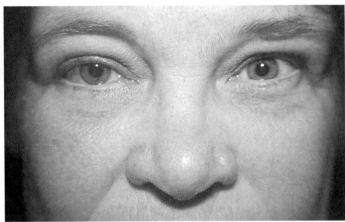

Figures 5–40 and 5–41   Preoperative and postoperative orbital decompression in the acute "wet" stage after intensive steroid therapy failed to prevent visual loss. Vision returned from hand motions to 20/40 postoperatively.

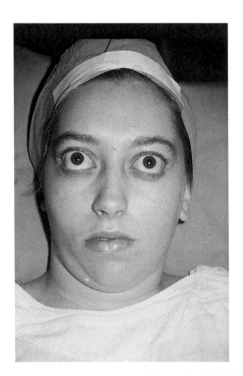

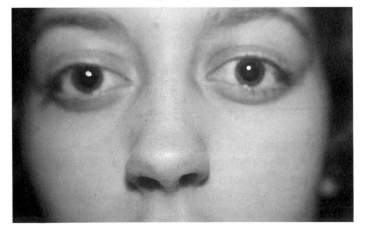

Figures 5–42, 5–43   Preoperative and postoperative orbital decompression.

of the globe (Fig. 5–41). On the other hand, with a long-standing exophthalmos, the ocular muscles and fascial connections may become so enlarged and fibrotic that even though the lateral and inferior walls of the orbit are removed, the socket formed by the infiltrated unyielding muscle cone and fascial bands does not mold to the expanded space but continues to hold the eye forward.

ORBITAL DECOMPRESSION TECHNIQUE (FIGS. 5–42 AND 5–43)

General anesthesia is required. We are indebted to Berke for his lateral canthal incision that replaced the disfiguring Krönlein approach for orbitotomy. The cornea is protected by a well-dampened piece of Gelfoam 1.5 × 1.5 cm, sutured to the conjunctiva. A 4 cm horizontal incision extending from the lateral canthus is made through skin, subcutaneous tissue, and muscle down to the orbital rim and lateral orbital wall (Fig. 5–44). The marked bleeding encountered is controlled by cautery. The conjunctiva is opened with scissors to the depth of the lateral cul-de-sac. An incision is made through the periosteum along the lateral orbital rim, and the lateral canthal ligament is severed by sharp dissection. The periosteum is freed from the bone with an elevator over the whole lateral wall both within the orbit and in the temporal fossa (Figs. 5–45 and 5–46).

The lateral orbital rim is more easily removed in small pieces than in one large section. A retractor is placed between the orbital periosteum and the bone to move the globe medially and protect it as the orbital rim is cut. The narrow blade of the Stryker bone saw is used to make two parallel cuts 2 cm apart through the heavy bone of the lateral rim (Fig. 5–47). This piece of bone is broken out with rongeurs, the vertical break being made where the heavy anterior rim joins the thin posterior plate (Figs. 5–48 and 5–49). Adequate retraction of the surrounding tissues is used while the remainder of the heavy bone of the lateral rim is removed with the saw in small slices, to the level of the zygoma below and to the superior orbital rim above. The orbital contents and fat bulge temporally. The thin posterior portion of the lateral wall is removed with rongeurs. The bleeding of the spongy bone at the posterior portion of the lateral wall can be controlled with bone wax. The wax is softened slightly to make it malleable, placed on a periosteal elevator, and forcibly pushed into the porous bone at the bleeding site. The exposed orbital periosteum and periorbita are cut away with great care. Pressure on the closed lid directed backward against the globe will cause the posterior structures to bulge into the defect in the lateral wall. The periosteum covering the temporal fossa is excised along with the tight fascial aponeurosis of the anterior portion of the temporalis muscle over the whole width of the area to be decompressed. If the aponeurosis of the temporalis muscle is not excised, it will restrict the lateral decompression of the orbital contents as much as if the bone had not been removed. A 3 cm portion of the muscle itself is excised to give adequate space for the decom-

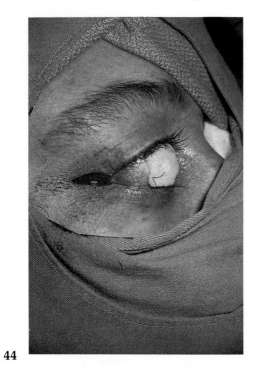

44

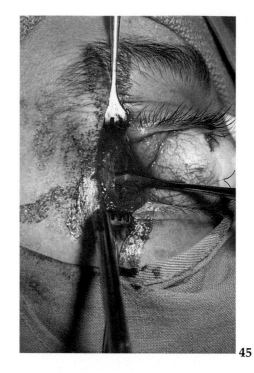

45

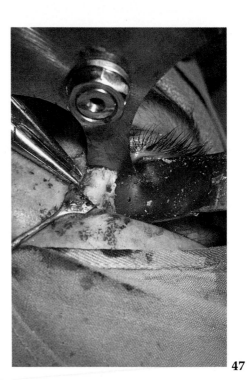

46

47

Figures 5–44 to 5–47

Figure 5–44   Incision extends from lateral canthus posteriorly
1¹/₂ to 2 cm.
Figures 5–45 and 5–46   Periosteum is stripped from the medial
and lateral aspects of the orbital rim.
Figure 5–47   A Stryker saw is used to cut the rim.

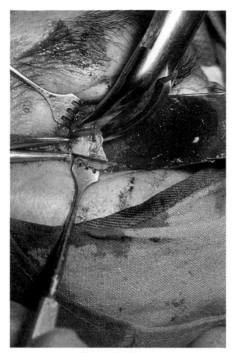

Figure 5–48

A rongeur is used to break out the rim following saw cuts.

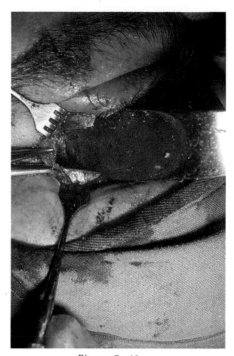

Figure 5–49

A 1.5 centimeter piece is removed initially.

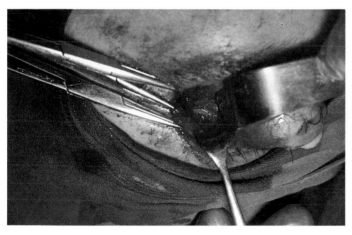

Figure 5–50

The orbital floor is exposed.

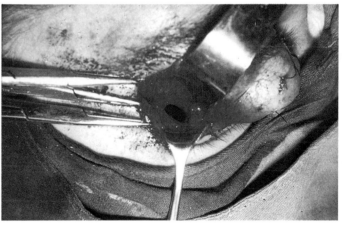

Figure 5–51

A hole is made in the orbital floor using chisel and sphenoid punch.

pression. This is best done with a cutting cautery to minimize bleeding. If more decompression is required, the floor of the orbit should be removed.

REMOVAL OF THE ORBITAL FLOOR

The skin of the lid and the orbicularis muscle are retracted inferiorly, and a spoon retractor is used to move the orbital contents upward and nasally (Fig. 5–50). The periosteum over the floor of the orbit is elevated and excised. A hole is made in the thin bone with hammer and chisel, and the whole lateral floor is removed with rongeurs (Fig. 5–51). An attempt is made to push the mucous membrane of the antrum downward to avoid injuring it; however, this is not always successful. The bony floor is removed nasally as far as the canal of the inferior orbital nerve, and the nerve is isolat-

161

ed before the nasal orbital floor is excised. In some instances, the nerve is inadvertently damaged, producing numbness of the skin and upper teeth for four to six months. It is necessary to excise the inferior fascia and periosteum to get the decompression into the antrum.

Irrigation of the whole field with gentamycin has been our policy. If bleeding has been marked and cannot be completely controlled, a ¼ inch Penrose drain is inserted deep into the temporal portion of the incision. (It can be removed after 24 hours.) The conjunctiva of the lateral cul-de-sac must be closed carefully with 7–0 chromic catgut buried sutures. One 4–0 chromic catgut suture in a mattress stitch is used to close the subcutaneous tissue at the lateral canthus, and occasionally another deep suture is placed in the subcutaneous tissue halfway along the incision. The skin is closed with 6–0 black silk sutures placed in a vertical mattress stitch at 4 mm intervals, interspaced with alternating 8–0 black silk sutures (Fig. 5–52). The orbit is dressed with a mild pressure bandage of two eye pads over the lids and one over the temporal incision. The anterior pads are held in place by elastic adhesive tape covered with regular adhesive tape. Minimal pressure is applied over the temporal incision.

The patient's immediate postoperative course on awakening is monitored for pain in the eye region. If it is marked, the nasal portion of the bandage is cut away for inspection of the cornea to check for visual disturbance, and the lateral dressing is watched for fresh bleeding. Should either occur, the dressings must be removed and the situation evaluated for a delayed deep bleed with a build-up of posterior orbital pressure. Fortunately, this has not happened in any of our patients, but it would require reopening the wound, evacuating the blood, and finding and cauterizing the bleeding point.

The globe does not "fly" back into the orbit as soon as the lateral and inferior walls are removed. It must be pushed back into the decompressed position by anterior-posterior pressure, with no pressure over the lateral incision. The anterior-posterior pressure must be firm but not so great as to cause occlusion of the retinal vessels. The correct pressure is, of course, a point of great importance, and the surgeon himself should apply the dressing, not the assistant surgeon or nurse.

The dressing should be changed in 24 hours and replaced by another mild anterior-posterior pressure dressing. Postoperative parenteral steroids should be given for one week and then tapered off. Systemic corticosteroids are often helpful for treatment of the acute congestion of the conjunctiva that may accompany thyroid disease (Figs. 5–53 and 5–54), but the progressive lid retraction, muscle imbalance and chronic exophthalmos are not, in general, affected by steroids and their use preoperatively offers no advantage.

Tarsorrhaphy

A lateral, paracentral, or medial tarsorrhaphy is the procedure of choice to prevent corneal exposure when lid closure is hampered

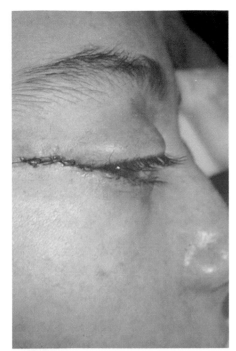

Figure 5–52

Fine skin closure leaves a very small scar.

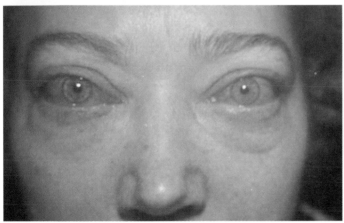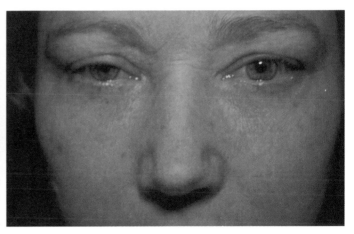

Figure 5–53 and 5–54

Before and after steroid therapy.

by thyroid disease, lid pathology, or seventh nerve palsy. Tarsor-rhaphies may be permanent or temporary and, therefore, should be done so they can be reopened at a later time without sacrifice of lid shape or function. In the case of a moribund patient who cannot be moved to an operating room, a simple tarsorrhaphy can be done at bedside. The marginal tarsorrhaphy is not meant to give permanent lid closure, but it is easy to do and can temporarily alleviate an exposure problem.

MARGINAL TARSORRHAPHY

The lid margins are denuded of epithelium temporally for the length of the desired tarsorrhaphy. Mattress sutures of 5–0 silk are used to suture the lids shut. The sutures are passed over cotton pledgets or silicone strips to prevent their cutting through the skin. The sutures extend from the skin 2 mm from the cilia line down through the gray line, then back through the gray line of the opposing lid to emerge from the skin again 2 mm from the lashes. These sutures are left in place ten days to two weeks. This is a temporary procedure, as in a short time contact areas usually stretch apart and either separate completely or become thin bands of epithelium that fail to keep the lids closed.

MODIFIED ELSCHNIG TARSORRHAPHY

A preferred and more reliable tarsorrhaphy is a variation of the Elschnig method that can be used as either a temporary or a permanent closure of the lids. The advantages of this procedure are that it can be a very effective permanent tarsorrhaphy and the lashes are not disturbed. If the tarsorrhaphy is opened, the lids resume their normal appearance. In the original procedure of Elschnig, tarsus was rotated from the lower to the upper lid. We rotate tarsus from the upper to the lower lids to avoid possible damage to the lacrimal ducts and because the larger piece of tarsus from the upper lid gives better support to the lower lid if ultimately the tarsorrhaphy is opened. The procedure is valuable in patients with very dry eyes for whom occlusion of the puncta and artificial tears have not been sufficient. It is also used for relief of exposure due to a seventh nerve palsy and in patients with thyroid exophthalmos, to reduce the exposure of the lateral scleral triangle.

Operative Technique. The skin of the lid and conjunctiva of the lateral half of the lid are injected with 1 per cent lidocaine (see p. 63). The upper lid is everted by two Adson forceps, one blade on conjunctiva and one on skin surface (Figs. 5–55 and 5–57). These are held by the assistant while the surgeon divides the lateral third or half of the tarsus into an anterior and posterior portion. The incision is made with a disposable Graefe knife along the openings of the meibomian glands. With the Adson forceps still holding the lid in the everted position, one blade of a straight scissors is inserted in the nasal end of the incision and a vertical cut is made in the posterior half of the tarsus to the retrotarsal margin (Figs. 5–56 and 5–58). This frees a lateral triangle of tissue, consisting of the posterior half of the tarsus covered on one side with conjunctiva (Fig. 5–59). The small strip of conjunctiva along the tarsal edge must be trimmed away to give a raw surface for good adherence when the flap is rotated into the corresponding defect to be made in the lower lid (Fig. 5–60).

The lower lid is everted in a similar manner, the tarsus split, and a triangle (corresponding to the size of the upper triangle) of the posterior half of the tarsus excised by making two cuts from the lid margin to join at the retrotarsal margin (Figs. 5–62 and 5–63).

Text continued on page 169

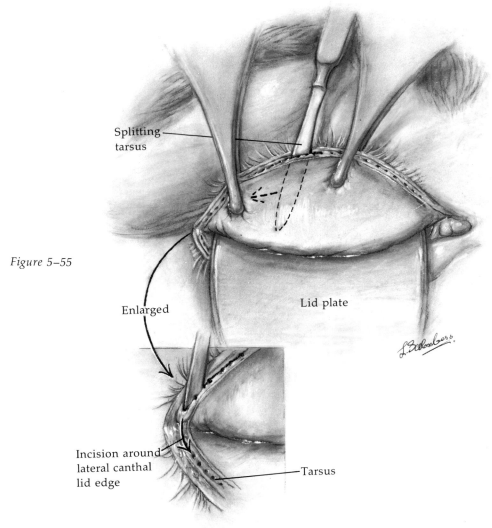

Splitting
tarsus

Lid plate

Figure 5–55

Enlarged

Incision around
lateral canthal
lid edge

Tarsus

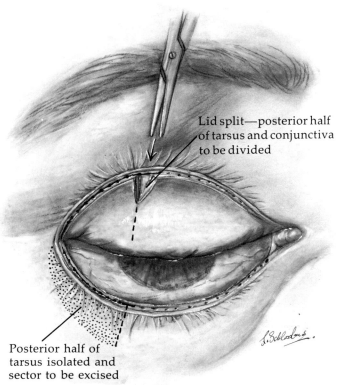

Lid split—posterior half
of tarsus and conjunctiva
to be divided

Figure 5–56

Posterior half of
tarsus isolated and
sector to be excised

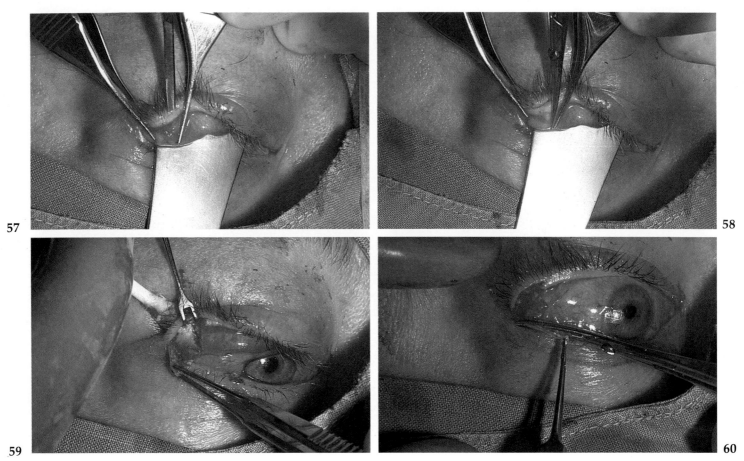

57

58

59

60

Figures 5–57 to 5–60

Figure 5–57 Tarsus is split with a disposable Graefe knife.
Figures 5–58 and 5–59   A triangle of the posterior portion of the tarsus is mobilized.
Figure 5–60   The conjunctiva at the lower edge of the triangle is excised.

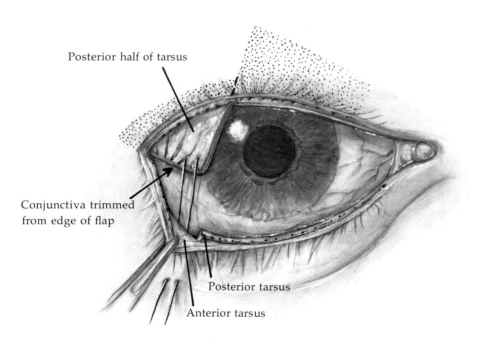

Posterior half of tarsus

Conjunctiva trimmed
from edge of flap

Posterior tarsus

Anterior tarsus

Figure 5–61

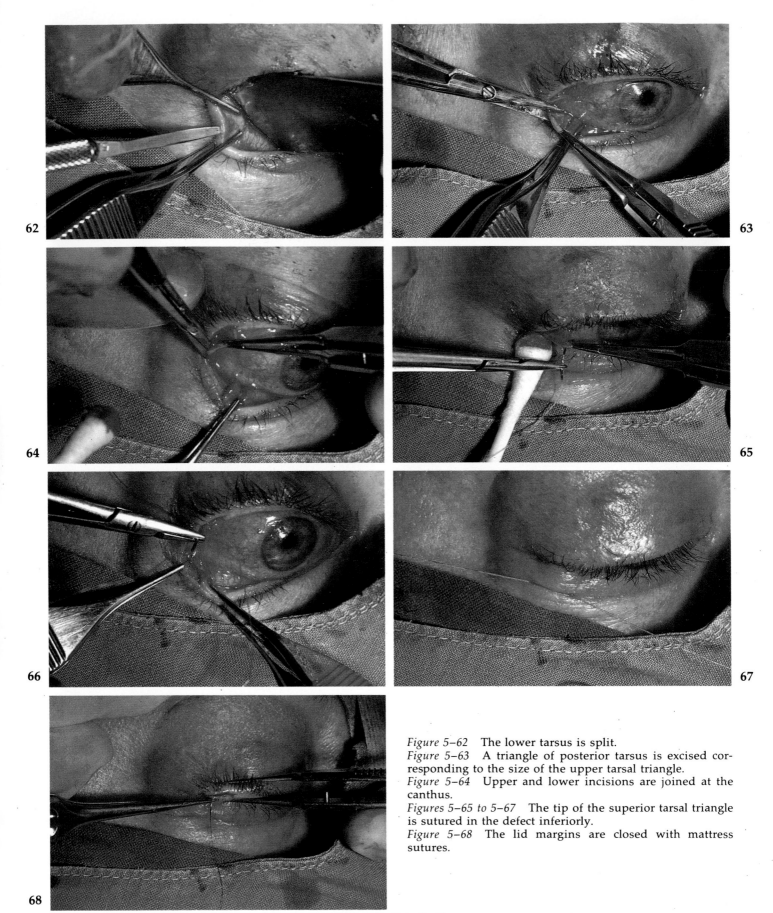

Figure 5–62   The lower tarsus is split.

Figure 5–63   A triangle of posterior tarsus is excised corresponding to the size of the upper tarsal triangle.

Figure 5–64   Upper and lower incisions are joined at the canthus.

Figures 5–65 to 5–67   The tip of the superior tarsal triangle is sutured in the defect inferiorly.

Figure 5–68   The lid margins are closed with mattress sutures.

Figures 5–62 to 5–68

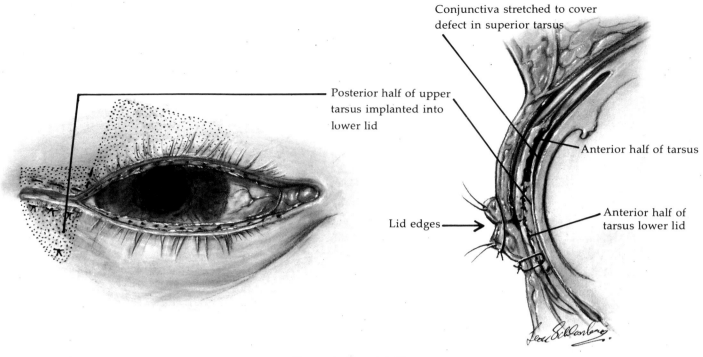

Posterior half of upper tarsus implanted into lower lid

Conjunctiva stretched to cover defect in superior tarsus

Anterior half of tarsus

Anterior half of tarsus lower lid

Lid edges

Figures 5–69 and 5–70

The incisions in the upper and lower lids must be joined at the lateral canthus (Fig. 5–64), otherwise, an epithelialized fistula will result that will constantly drain tears and cause skin irritation.

A double-armed, 5–0 suture is passed through the nasal tip of the superior tarsal triangle and then to the apex of the inferior excised triangle (Figs. 5–61, 5–65, 5–66). The needles are passed through the skin of the lid and tied (Figs. 5–67 and 5–69). This firmly rotates the upper tarsal triangle into the lower lid defect. The edges of the lids are sutured together with mattress stitches of 8–0 black silk, everting the edges so the raw surfaces will come in contact and adhere (Figs. 5–68 and 5–70). The sutures are removed in one week.

Opening a Tarsorrhaphy

When a tarsorrhaphy is opened, the incision is made with straight scissors just beneath the lash line of the upper lid, which has not been disturbed. This is done under local anesthesia; 2 to 3 cc of injection on each side of the proposed line of incision is required to give complete anesthesia. The raw areas between the conjunctiva and epithelium of the anterior lid margin are not closed with sutures but are permitted to epithelialize and re-form the normal gray line. Suturing these edges may rotate the cilia line inward and cause corneal abrasion.

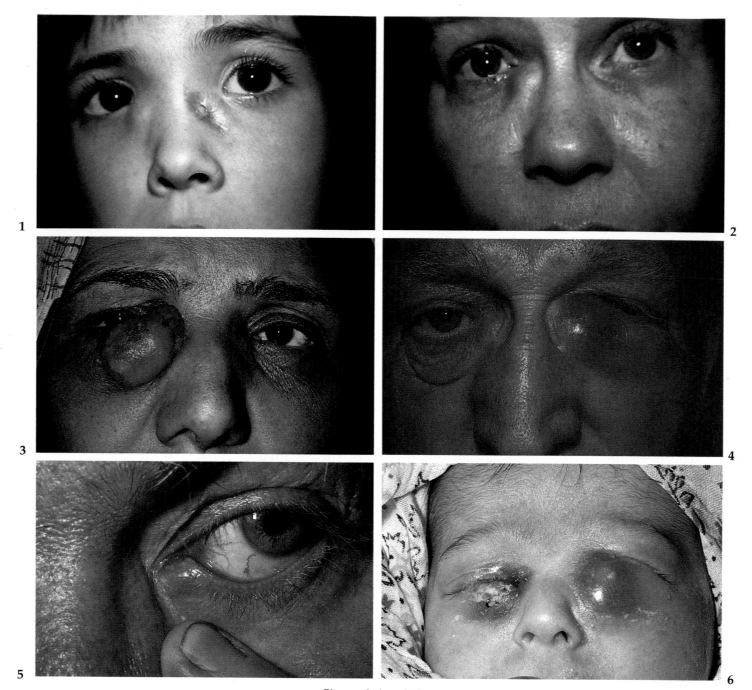

Figures 6–1 to 6–6

Figure 6–1 Recurrent dacryocystitis repeatedly treated incorrectly by incision and drainage.
Figure 6–2 Chronic dacryocystitis.
Figure 6–3 and 6–4 Acute dacryocystitis.
Figure 6–5 Infection of canalicular ampulla.
Figure 6–6 Bilateral acute dacryocystitis beginning at age two days. Treatment with systemic antibiotics and warm compresses led to spontaneous drainage and resolution of infection.

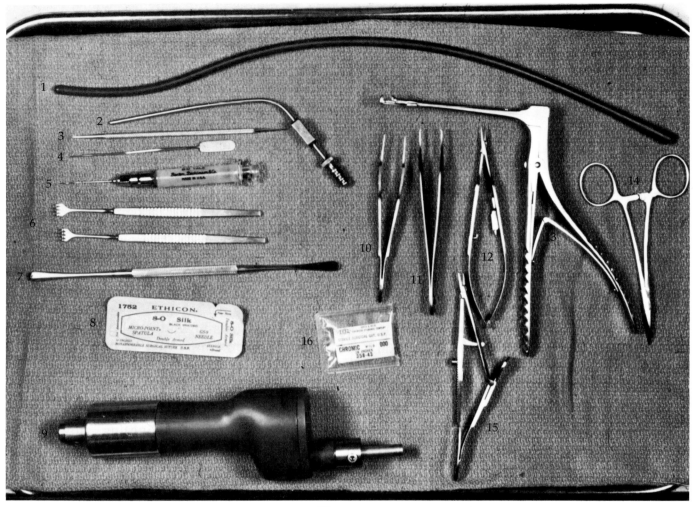

Figure 6–7

1. Rubber catheter
2. Small suction tip
3. Punctum dilator
4. Olive tipped lacrimal probe
5. Lacrimal irrigating syringe
6. Skin rakes
7. Freer elevator
8. Skin suture

9. Stryker lacrimal trephine
10. Fine forceps
11. Adson forceps
12. Fine needle holder
13. Sphenoid punch
14. Fine curved hemostat
15. Regular needle holder
16. Lacrimal suture

tears into the nose. If spontaneous reopening does not occur within 6 months, probing is necessary. If the blockage is complicated by infection, antibiotics should be used, and probing should be done as soon as the baby is a good anesthetic risk. Infection is rare before the age of 1 month; however, it does occur (Fig. 6–6) and should be treated with hot compresses and antibiotics.

The probing procedure consists of breaking the delicate mucous membrane block at the nasal orifice of the tract. Unfortunately, probing has been considered by some a procedure of such minor importance that it requires little surgical skill, and on some ophthalmologic services it has been delegated to a junior physician, often with disastrous results. A common cause of chronic dacryocystitis is such unskilled attempts. The lining of the lacrimal tract has the same friability as the conjunctiva, and damage is easily produced even with a blunt instrument. The healing of an injury in-

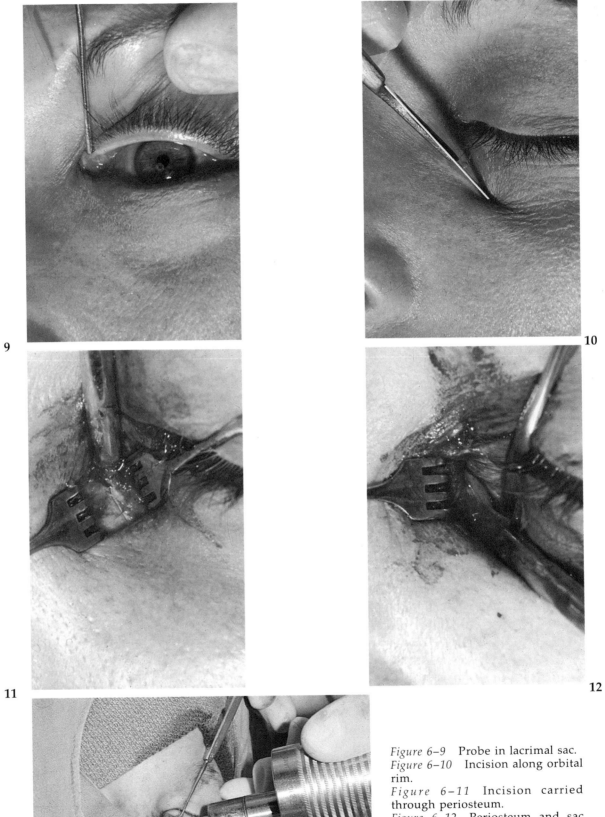

9

10

11

12

13

Figure 6-9   Probe in lacrimal sac.
Figure 6-10   Incision along orbital rim.
Figure 6-11   Incision carried through periosteum.
Figure 6-12   Periosteum and sac are retracted from lacrimal fossa.
Figure 6-13   7 mm. Iliff trephine and Stryker handle is applied to lacrimal crest.

Figure 6-9 to 6-13

178

sion, which extends 2 cm from the medial canthal ligament along the rim. A bold incision to the orbital rim (Fig. 6–10) is made with a No. 15 Bard-Parker knife through skin, subcutaneous tissue, orbicularis muscle, and periosteum. This incision should be placed in the normal skin fold for the best cosmetic result. The reason for insisting on this single bold cut down to the periosteum is that layer-by-layer dissection will often cause the tissues to slide on one another as they are retracted by the assistant, and the direct course to the orbital crest is thus lost. This makes the surgery exceedingly difficult, especially if severe bleeding occurs. The incision over the anterior lacrimal crest is located in the thin skin of the lids, and postoperative scarring is practically nonexistent. We believe that placing the initial incision closer to the nose, as advocated by some surgeons to reduce the bleeding, is not valid. Also, the scar of a more nasally placed incision is more likely to show postoperatively than one in a normal lid crease along the anterior lacrimal crest.

Skin rake retractors (Blair) provide adequate exposure of the anterior lacrimal crest (Fig. 6–11) and have proved more satisfactory than a speculum, because the retractors can be easily adjusted to control superficial bleeders. The operative field is kept dry by suction, and blood vessels are occluded with cautery.

If the incision of the periosteum along the lacrimal crest has not been complete with the first through-and-through cut, it is deepened to bone with the Bard-Parker knife. A periosteal elevator (Freer) is used to strip the periosteum and sac (to which it is closely adherent) from the bony lacrimal fossa. These tissues are retracted together, thus exposing the anterior lacrimal crest and fossa (Fig. 6–12).

The dacryotrephine of the Stryker saw is placed straddling the anterior crest (Figs. 6–13 and 6–14) and is directed nasally, inferiorly, and slightly posteriorly. Slight rotation of the saw increases the cutting action. The bone is cut cleanly, and the plug usually comes out as the trephine blade is withdrawn; if not, it is freed with a periosteal elevator and removed with forceps (Figs. 6–15 and 6–16). Bone wax provides adequate control of any bone bleeding.

Usually the 7 mm trephine hole must be enlarged with a sphenoid punch to provide a more direct passage for the catheter from the nose to the neck of the sac. Any spicules of bone can be removed easily with the punch, and the hole can be enlarged to give a more elliptical opening, the extension being made downward.

A cruciate or H-shaped incision is made in the nasal mucous membrane if it is normal in thickness. If there is marked hypertrophy of the mucous membrane, it is completely excised over the trephine opening (Fig. 6–17).

Often, hypertrophic mucous membrane of the nose will bleed profusely; therefore, by shifting the suction from the operative incision to the nose at the site of the internal opening, the surgical field can be kept dry, and the suction tube will not obscure the work area.

A probe is re-passed into the sac, usually through the upper punctum. The end of the probe in the sac helps to identify exactly the nasal wall of the sac, which is opened with a No. 11 Bard-

179

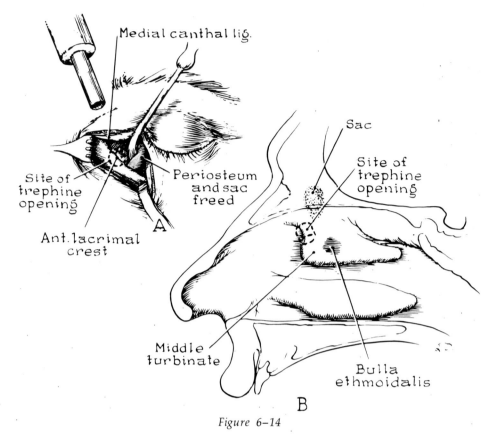

Figure 6–14

Diagram showing where the trephine opening enters the nose.

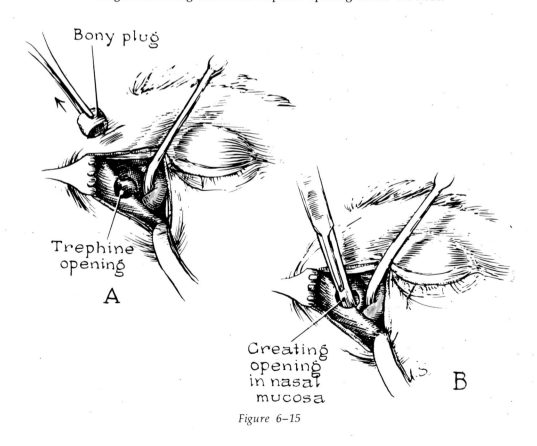

Figure 6–15

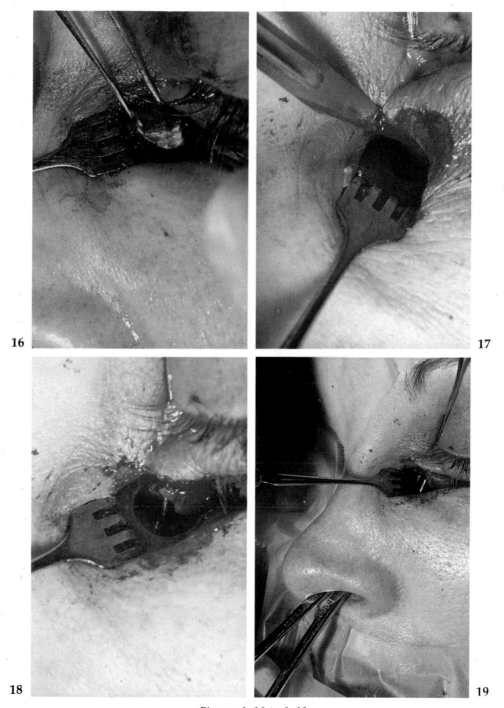

Figures 6–16 to 6–19

Figure 6–16 Bone plug removed.
Figure 6–17 Nasal mucosa is opened.
Figure 6–18 A probe through the upper canaliculus emerges through the opened sac.
Figure 6–19 Small curved hemostat is passed up the nose; here is shown at the bony orifice touching the end of the probe in the sac.

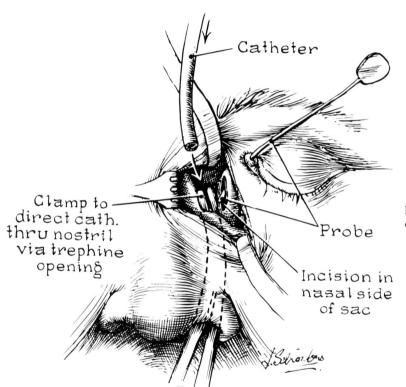

Catheter

Clamp to
direct cath.
thru nostril
via trephine
opening

Probe

Incision in
nasal side
of sac

Figure 6–20

Diagram of passing catheter into the nose by
catching the end with the Halsted clamp.

Parker knife with a vertical incision to expose the end of the probe (Fig. 6–18).

A curved Halsted clamp (Figs. 6–19 and 6–20) is passed up through the nose into the nasal trephine window to grasp the tip of a catheter, which is then drawn into the nose and out the external nares. The proximal end of the catheter is cut off, leaving 3 cm projecting from the wound.

A double-armed, 3–0 chromic catgut suture with a small, half-curved, special needle (Ethicon No. 748–G) is placed through the wall of the catheter, 1 cm from the cut end (Figs. 6–21 and 6–25). This end of the catheter is grasped with toothed forceps and is pushed gently into the wound past the end of the probe and then is pulled back, threading the catheter over the lacrimal probe that is lying in the sac (Figs. 6–22 and 6–26). Tension on the suture pulls the catheter up into the neck of the sac, with the probe acting as a guide. Care is taken that the cut edges of the sac wall are not caught on the end of the catheter, but lie around it (Figs. 6–23 and 6–27).

The two arms of the suture are then passed through the anterior sac wall and subcutaneous tissue, and as they are being pulled tight and tied, the catheter is forced into the neck of the sac. Placing the suture 1 cm from the end of the catheter (as mentioned) is important in producing this effect.

The probe is then withdrawn, and as the skin rakes are removed, the tissues fall together and the catheter acts as a splint. The cut edges of the medial wall of the sac and the cut edges of the nasal mucous membrane are in contact. Slight tension on the catheter, after it is fastened to the ala of the nose with the 3–0 chromic catgut suture, enhances this tissue approximation and the catheter splinting action.

The skin of the incision is closed with 8–0 interrupted but closely placed silk sutures (Figs. 6–24 and 6–28) and the wound is lightly dressed with a nonadherent dressing and an eye pad.

The patient is hospitalized for only 24 hours. The skin sutures are removed after 4 days. The catheter is removed at 10 days by cutting the suture in the ala and giving a short quick tug on the catheter, thus breaking the now friable catgut suture between the catheter and the anterior sac wall.

PREVENTION AND MANAGEMENT OF
COMPLICATIONS

Incision of the skin, subcutaneous tissue, and periosteum by steps is not as satisfactory as the through-and-through incision, with immediate retraction of the wound edges by rake retractors. When a stepwise incision is used, the tissues tend to slide, and the operator may miss the anterior crest, thereby cutting into the sac or going too far toward the nose. The canthal ligament must not be cut, since nothing is gained by exposing the underlying area and such cutting produces a cosmetic deformity. The slightly curved incision following the orbital rim lies in a skin fold, and the resulting scar disappears within 3 months.

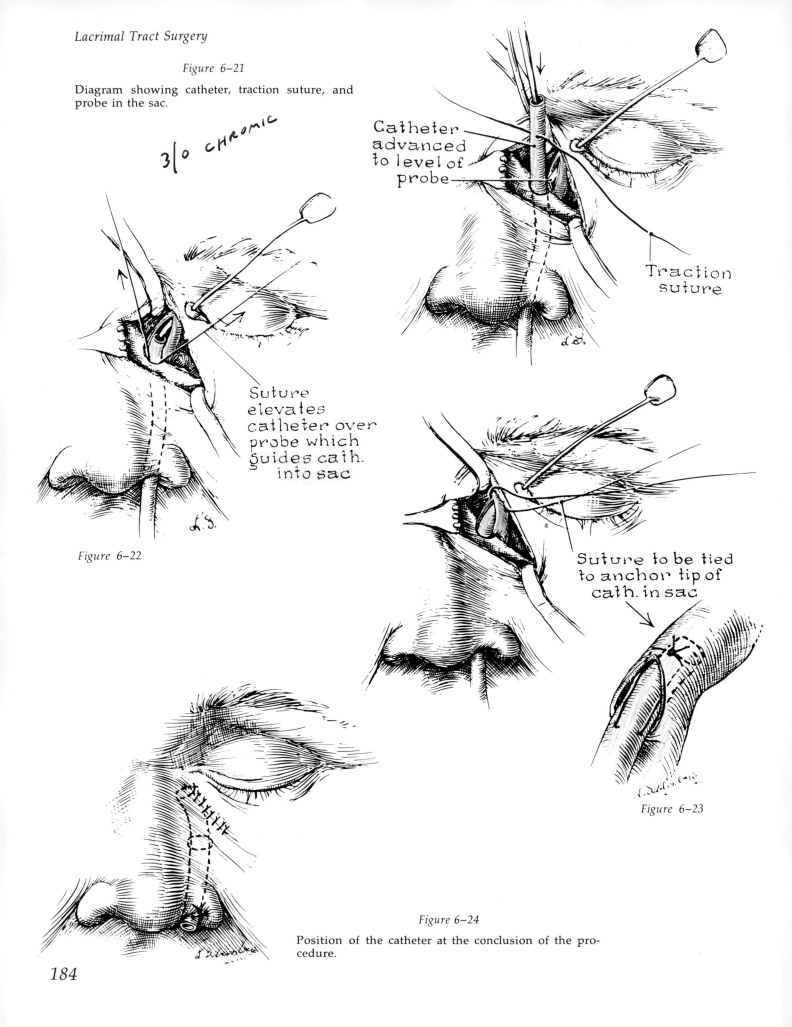

Figure 6–21

Diagram showing catheter, traction suture, and probe in the sac.

3/0 CHROMIC

Catheter advanced to level of probe

Traction suture

Suture elevates catheter over probe which guides cath. into sac

Figure 6–22

Suture to be tied to anchor tip of cath. in sac

Figure 6–23

Figure 6–24

Position of the catheter at the conclusion of the procedure.

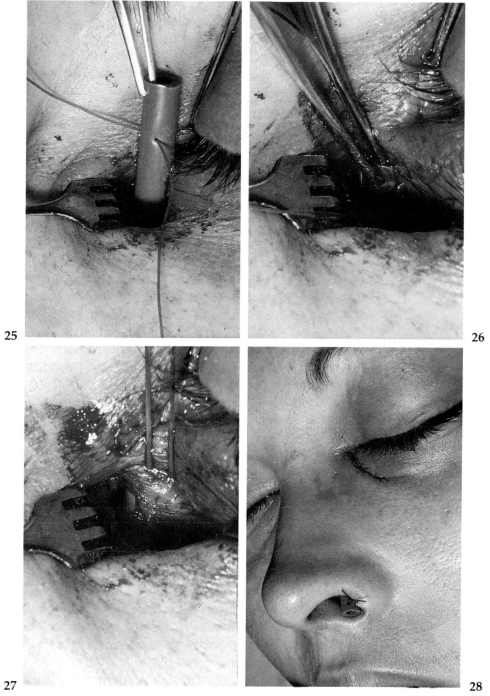

25 26

27 28

Figures 6–24 to 6–27

Figure 6–25 Catheter pulled through the opening into the nose. A 3–0 chromic suture is placed 1 cm. from the catheter end.
Figure 6–26 Catheter is passed over the lacrimal probe in the neck of the sac.
Figure 6–27 Suture is brought through the anterior sac wall.
Figure 6–28 Closure.

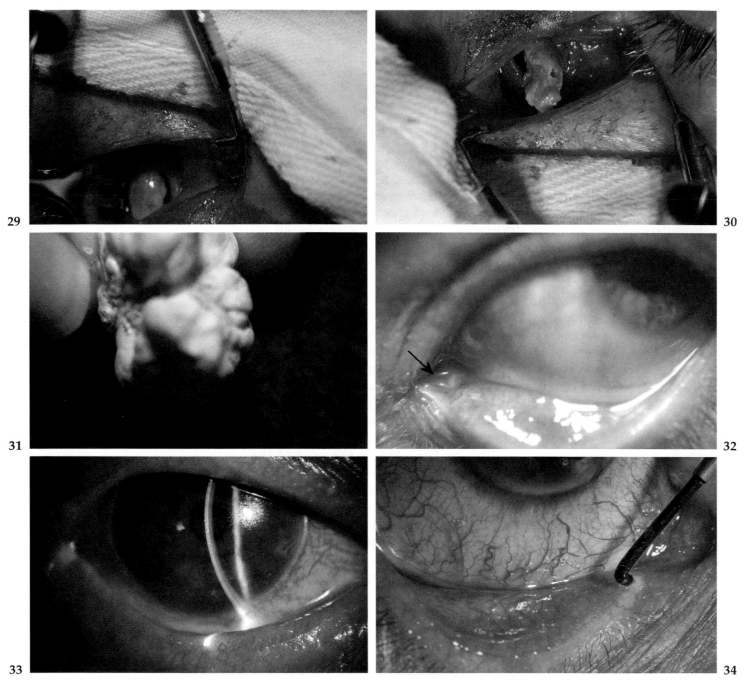

Figures 6–29 to 6–34

Figure 6–29 Lacrimal stone in opened sac.
Figure 6–30 Holes in dacryolith caused by probing.
Figure 6–31 Osteoma in ethmoid area impinging on lacrimal sac caused dacryocystitis.
Figure 6–32 Proper Jones tube placement.
Figure 6–33 Keratitis sicca.
Figure 6–34 Punctal occlusion.

beneath the plica toward the nose, and downward at an angle that enters the nasal ostium. Into this tract is slipped the Jones or Reinecke tube. The Jones tube should be long enough to enter the nose but not touch the septum. The Reinecke tube is formed so that the lower end of the tube lies in the nose. The upper end of the tube is fastened to the conjunctiva beneath the plica with a 6–0 nylon suture. In the case of the Reinecke tube, an actual suture bite in the plastic can be taken. The object of this suture is to keep the conjunctiva from folding over and closing the tube. It is possible to trim the end of the Reinecke tube if it touches or irritates the globe. If a Jones tube causes irritation, it can be replaced with a shorter tube.

In time, usually about a year, the tube will guide the establishment of an epithelialized conjunctivonasal mucous membrane tract, and the tube can then be removed.

The tube can be kept patent by having the patient hold the nose and breathe in. Tubes sometimes become occluded with a clot or mucus and must be irrigated — or removed, cleaned, and replaced. This is not a difficult procedure and can be done during an office visit.

Congenital Lacrimal Fistulas

Congenital lacrimal fistulas from the sac to the skin (Fig. 6–35) are rare. They produce a tear drop that wets the skin. In addition to being annoying, this can cause skin irritation. Cauterizing the tract or closing the skin opening is usually unsuccessful. We have closed these fistulas by passing a fine probe down the tract. An 8–0 silk purse-string suture is placed in the skin around the probe and is tied tightly (Fig. 6–36). Slight traction is made on the probe as the tract is being dissected free from the surrounding tissue for its total length. A deep 7–0 chromic suture is placed at the sac level, and the skin is closed with an 8–0 black silk suture (Fig. 6–37).

DRY EYE SYNDROME

One of the most commonly missed causes of ocular discomfort is the partially dry eye (Fig. 6–33). It occurs more frequently in women than in men and is often associated with dryness of the other mucous membranes. Symptoms may be itching, burning, general ocular irritation with some chronic infection of the conjunctiva, and occasionally photophobia. These patients have a reduced Schirmer test — less than 5 mm in 5 minutes. In spite of this, their chief complaint may be a feeling of excess of tears or a "watery" eye. This sensation is caused by an accumulation of mucoid material and debris that may at times blur the vision.

Examination of the eye usually shows a moderate or large amount of cellular debris on the cornea and in the cul-de-sacs. The cornea will often stain with fluorescein or rose bengal solution, and there may be typical epithelial filaments hanging on the cornea.

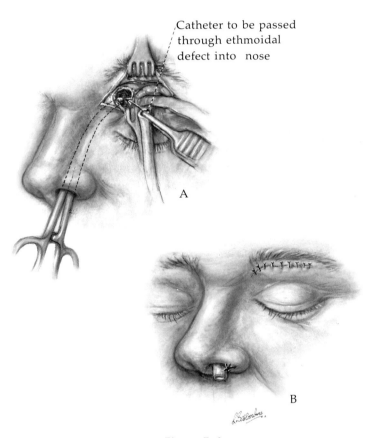

Catheter to be passed
through ethmoidal
defect into nose

A

B

Figure 7–9

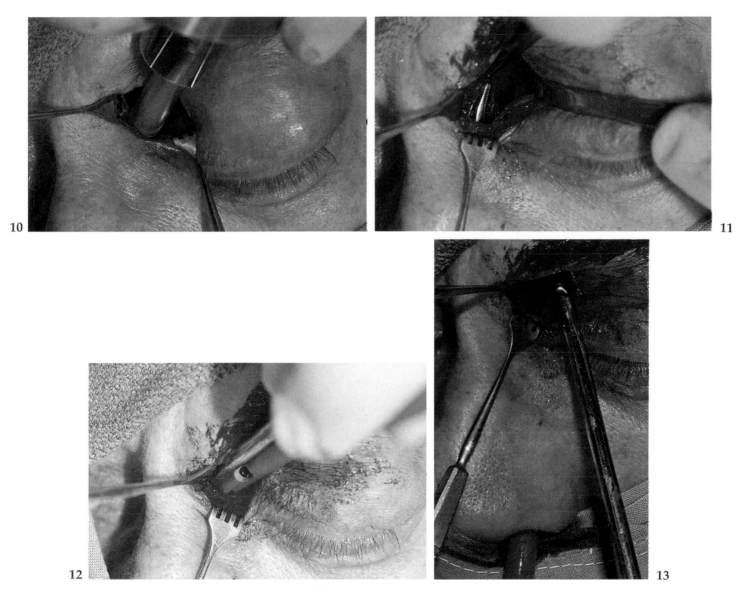

Figures 7–10 to 7–13

Figure 7–10   7 mm trephine is used to open into the nose.
Figure 7–11   A curved hemostat is passed up the nasal passage through the trephine opening.
Figure 7–12   The hemostat is used to pass a red rubber catheter from the sinus down through the nose.
Figure 7–13   The position of the catheter is such that the upper end lies in the frontal sinus.

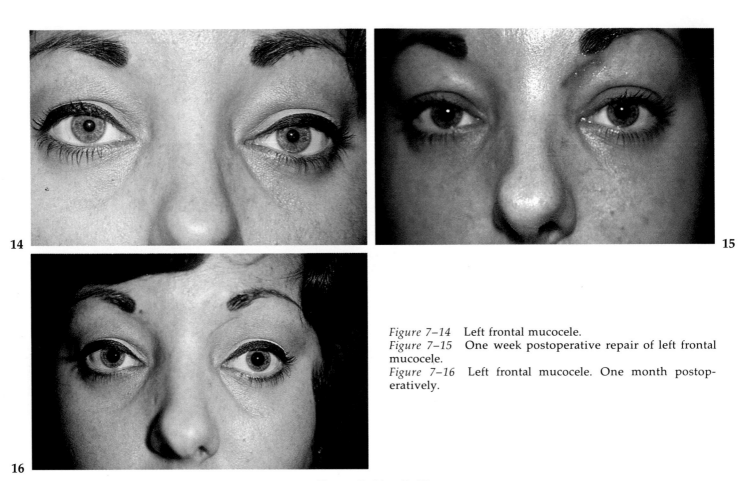

Figure 7–14   Left frontal mucocele.
Figure 7–15   One week postoperative repair of left frontal mucocele.
Figure 7–16   Left frontal mucocele. One month postoperatively.

Figures 7–14 to 7–17

cosmetic defect follows the operation (Figs. 7–14, 7–15, and 7–16), and any slight postoperative muscle imbalance returns to normal quite promptly.

Some otolaryngologists have criticized this procedure, indicating that with this method the sinus is not ablated as it is when it is packed with fat, muscle, or the bone of the frontal plate. It must be understood that our method does not attempt to destroy the sinus but merely to establish adequate drainage — the lack of which was the cause of the original problem. We wish to point out that mucoceles and infections of the antrum, ethmoid, and sphenoid sinuses are handled by otolaryngologists by establishing adequate drainage, so our method, which has proven successful, is not an unusual solution to the problem. Dr. J. Lawton Smith has noted the occurrence of sinus carcinoma in several mucoceles and has emphasized that histologic examination of the removed epithelium should be done.*

Figure 7–17 is a preoperative x-ray demonstrating a defect in the roof of the left orbit. Figure 7–18 shows the same patient 1 year postoperatively. The orbital roof has been reformed, and the sinus is well drained and clear.

---

*Smith, J. L.: Wilmer Residents Association Meeting, 1975.

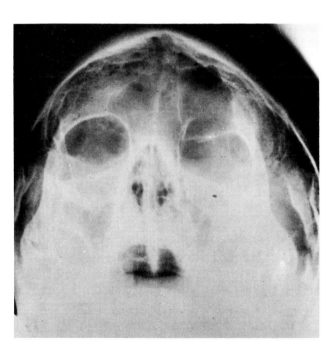

Figure 7–17

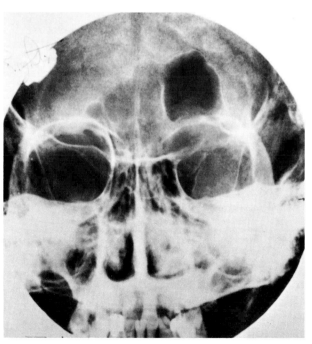

Figure 7–18

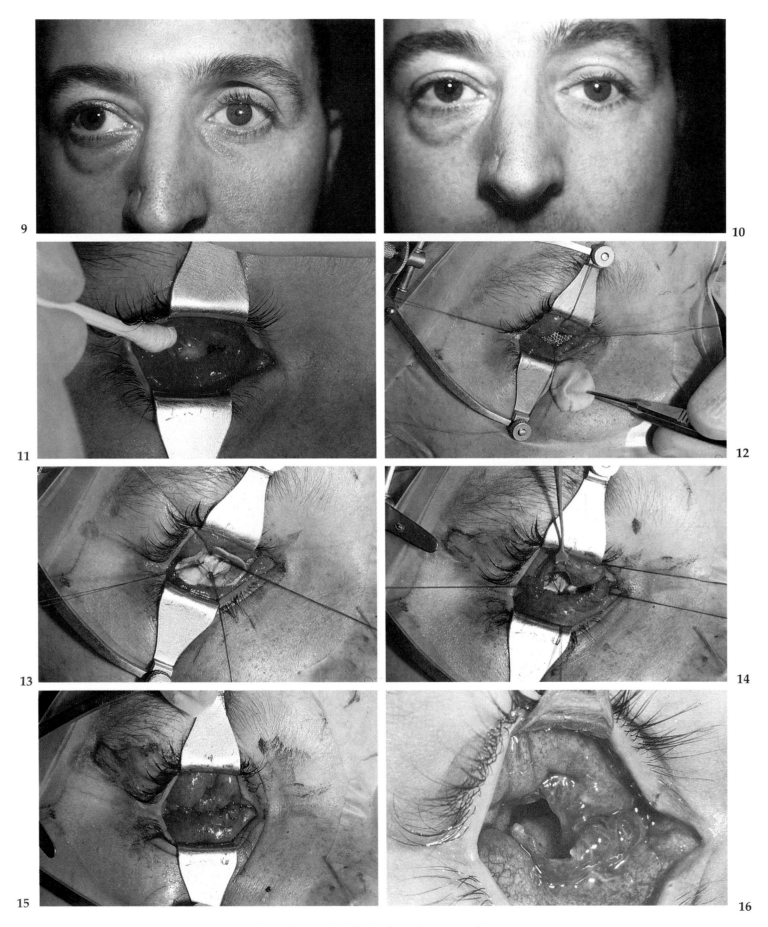

9

10

11

12

13

14

15

16

210   *Figures 8–9 to 8–16   See legends on opposite page.*

The Extruded Implant

If a portion of an implant becomes exposed shortly after enucleation (Fig. 8–11), it will in most cases eventually be extruded unless preventive measures are taken immediately. It is possible to reinforce the conjunctiva and Tenon's capsule by using a piece of preserved sclera to prevent further extrusion.

TECHNIQUE: COVERING A PARTIALLY
EXTRUDED IMPLANT WITH A CAP OF
PRESERVED SCLERA

General anesthesia is necessary because bleeding is usually marked, and adequate local anesthesia is difficult to maintain.

The conjunctiva and Tenon's capsule are dissected from the implant as far back as the equator. A cap of preserved sclera is cut to cover the face of the implant (Fig. 8–12). Four double-armed 4–0 absorbable sutures are passed through Tenon's capsule in the region of the four rectus muscles at the base of the dissection, brought out through the sclera, and tied (Fig. 8–13). Two arms are then passed back through Tenon's capsule deep in the dissection and brought out through the conjunctiva in the cul-de-sacs and again tied (Fig. 8–14). This puts tension on the scleral cap against the implant. Tenon's capsule is closed with a purse-string 4–0 absorbable suture, and the conjunctiva is closed with interrupted stitches of 6–0 chromic catgut (Fig. 8–15).

If the implant has been exposed for many months, its bed becomes lined with epithelium and harbors a low-grade infection (Fig. 8–16). When this has taken place we have not been successful in closing the anterior defect in Tenon's capsule and conjunctiva with a scleral patch; instead, we have developed the brow approach. An inflatable silicone sphere is inserted through a brow incision into the muscle cone. A sterile field can be maintained because the infected conjunctiva is not opened. The invaginated epithelium-lined socket of the original implant is pushed forward as the sphere is inflated and helps form the new socket.

TECHNIQUE: BROW APPROACH TO REPLACE
AN EXTRUDED IMPLANT

A 3 cm incision is made (Fig. 8–17) in the lateral brow just below the cilia line — through the skin, subcutaneous tissue, and orbicularis muscle — down through the periosteum at the dependent edge of the superior orbital rim (Fig. 8–18). Using a Freer elevator, the periosteum is easily separated from bone of the superotemporal portion of the orbit (Fig. 8–19). An anterior-posterior incision

---

Figures 8–9 to 8–16

Figures 8–9 to 8–10   Pre and postoperative repair by insertion of an inflatable sphere of a sunken socket due to absorption of orbital fat.
Figure 8–11   Exposure of an orbital implant.
Figures 8–12 to 8–15   Preserved sclera is sutured to Tenon's capsule and is covered by conjunctiva.
Figure 8–16   Conjunctival epithelial ingrowth surrounds an implant if it is exposed for an extended length of time.

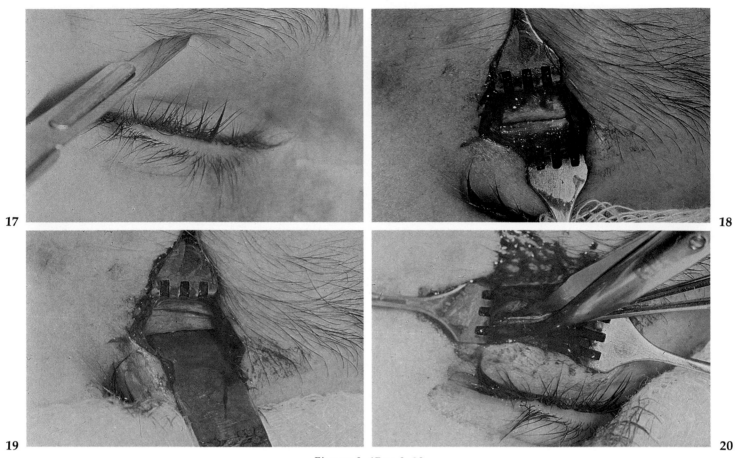

17 18
19 20

Figures 8–17 to 8–20

Figures 8–17 and 8–18   A brow incision is carried down through the periosteum.
Figure 8–19   The periosteum is elevated from the orbital rim.
Figure 8–20   Periosteum opened in anterior-posterior direction.

is then made in the periosteum, perpendicular to the original incision and at its midpoint, and is extended back into the orbit for approximately 2.5 cm (Fig. 8–20). The lacrimal gland and lateral rectus muscle are temporal to this incision; the frontal nerve, levator muscle, and superior rectus muscle are nasal. These important structures are not damaged.

A curved hemostat is used by blunt dissection to open the orbital fat (Fig. 8–21) and to make a pocket in the muscle cone of sufficient size for the insertion of a silicone sphere. This pocket should be enlarged inferiorly so that the inflated sphere will tend to stay in the muscle cone rather than ride up along the entrance tract. Should it move back up the tract, it would interfere with the lid motion and might produce a ptosis.

The silicone sphere, 16 or 18 mm in diameter, is collapsed by extracting the air with a 30-gauge needle on a syringe inserted through a special thickened area in the wall of the sphere (Fig. 8–22). While held collapsed with a clamp, the sphere is inserted through the tract of the prepared pocket in the muscle cone (Fig. 8–23). The needle remains in place in the collapsed sphere as it is being inserted. When the sphere has been properly placed, it is refilled with air and the needle is withdrawn (Fig. 8–24).

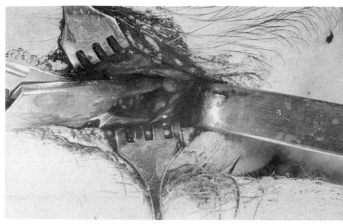

21

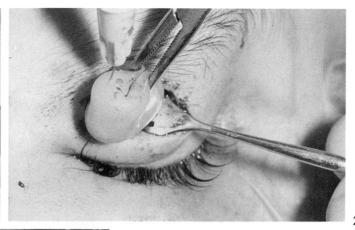

22

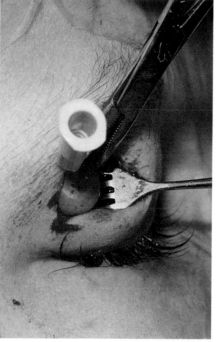

23

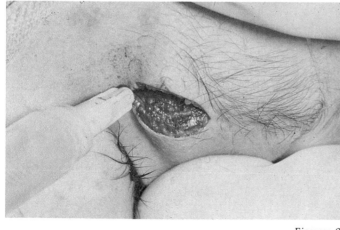

24

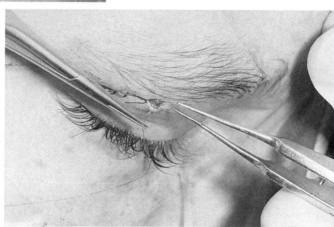

25

Figures 8–21 to 8–25

Figure 8–21   A pocket is made in the muscle cone.
Figures 8–22 and 8–23   Insertion of the collapsed sphere.
Figure 8–24   The sphere is reinflated.
Figure 8–25   Closure.

After the sphere is in place, 5–0 chromic catgut is used to close the tract of insertion so that the implant cannot migrate. Catgut is also used to close the anterior-posterior and brow incisions of the periosteum. The subcutaneous tissues usually fall into place without suturing but the skin is closed with interrupted 8–0 black silk (Fig. 8–25). A conformer is placed in the socket, and mild pressure dressing is applied. A prosthesis can be fitted in three weeks (Figs. 8–26 and 8–27).

Symblephara

Symblephara between the lids and the globe may completely obliterate the cul-de-sacs. This is seen in Stevens-Johnson disease and after chemical burns, and repair may require many mucous membrane grafts. It is quite difficult to get enough mucous membrane from the lip or cheek at one operation to re-form both the upper and lower cul-de-sacs, so usually the lower one is re-formed first and the upper is done at a later date.

TECHNIQUE: MUCOUS MEMBRANE GRAFT TO THE CUL-DE-SAC

General anesthesia is required.

OBTAINING THE GRAFT

We have had difficulty getting a large enough piece of mucous membrane with the mucotome, so we routinely use free-hand removal of a full thickness section. The lower lip is put on stretch, and the large lip clamp (Storz No. E-2965) applied. As the clamp is rotated downward, the mucous membrane is stretched. With a No. 15 Bard-Parker blade a rectangle of mucous membrane, as large as can be cut with the clamp in place, is marked out lightly. A 6–0 black silk suture is placed in each corner of the rectangle, and the graft is carefully undermined with sharp and blunt dissection. An occasional small perforation occurs, but this does no harm. The graft is pinned on a teak board and all fatty tissue removed.

Immediate bleeding from the graft site on the lip is controlled by a gauze pack. Surprisingly little postoperative discomfort is experienced and the only care needed is a liquid diet for the first 2 or 3 days.

INSERTING THE GRAFT

If any usable conjunctiva remains, it should be carefully preserved. Figure 8–28 shows a patient with Stevens-Johnson disease who had no conjunctiva available.

The lower lid is separated from the globe, and bleeding is controlled with cautery. The eye is rotated upward as far as possible, and the lid is everted on a Desmarres retractor to bare the depths of

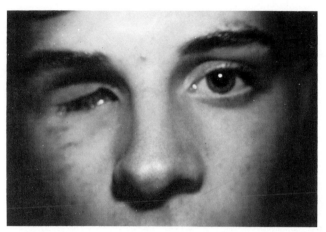

Figure 8–26

Three attempts at replacement of the extruded implant through the conjunctiva had failed.

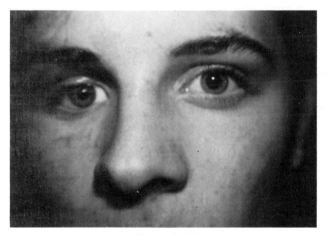

Figure 8–27

Postoperative insertion of inflatable implant through the brow.

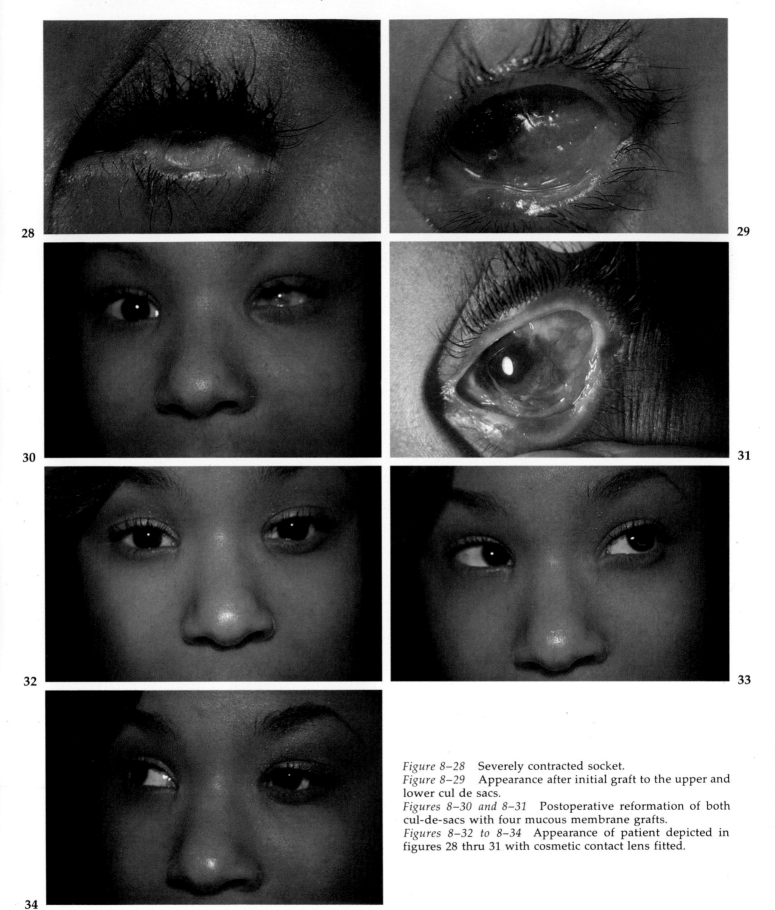

Figure 8–28   Severely contracted socket.
Figure 8–29   Appearance after initial graft to the upper and lower cul de sacs.
Figures 8–30 and 8–31   Postoperative reformation of both cul-de-sacs with four mucous membrane grafts.
Figures 8–32 to 8–34   Appearance of patient depicted in figures 28 thru 31 with cosmetic contact lens fitted.

Figures 8–28 to 8–34

the dissected cul-de-sac. The graft is folded, and three double-armed 6–0 black silk sutures are used to secure the fold deep in the cul-de-sac. The two ends of each suture are passed near to or through the periosteum of the orbital rim and brought out to the skin and tied. In some instances it is helpful to pass the sutures through a strip of silicone that will produce the fold in the graft. These sutures fix the folded graft as deep in the cul-de-sac as possible. The free edges are now sutured to the lid margin and to the remaining conjunctival edge with 7–0 chromic catgut sutures. If a small area of bare sclera should remain, it will epithelialize.

Suture lines of the graft should not be allowed to come into contact, for they may adhere. The graft must be positioned so the suture lines on the globe and on the lid are not juxtaposed. This is done by dissecting as much conjunctiva as possible from the lid so that it can rotate posteriorly to cover the globe. The graft can then be positioned primarily on the palpebral surface. It is important that a bare area of the globe and a bare area of the lid not come in contact because another symblepharon will form. No ointment is used at the close of operation, but the eye is dressed with Decadron ointment on the second day.

Several months later, a similar procedure is done on the upper cul-de-sac (Fig. 8–29) Multiple grafts are often necessary. Four such procedures were necessary in the case presented here. Each case offers its own special problem, but perseverance and care can produce a satisfactory result. Figures 8–32 to 8–34 demonstrate the final appearance of the patient shown in Figures 8–28 to 8–31. After the formation of adequate cul-de-sacs, a cosmetic scleral contact lens was fitted.

Contracted Sockets

SLIGHTLY CONTRACTED SOCKETS

In patients in whom the globe has been removed and an implant either was not inserted or has extruded, the socket may become contracted as a result of scarring (Fig. 8–35). The scarred orbital contents and the deep contracting bands can be removed through a brow incision. The socket can then be packed with sea sponges to stretch the remaining conjunctiva.

This approach through a lateral brow incision is exactly the same as for the insertion of an inflatable sphere after an implant has been extruded. The anterior portions of the extraocular muscles that are bound to the central mass of scar tissue (Fig. 8–36) and the associated fat are removed by sharp dissection, taking special care that the conjunctiva of the socket is not opened. Bands of scar tissue immediately behind the conjunctiva can be located by palpating with a finger in the socket. The adequate exposure through the brow incision permits these bands to be picked up and excised. As the bands are cut, the conjunctival sac becomes enlarged, the tenting disappears, and the tissue folds can be spread out so that the conjunctiva becomes paper thin as it is stretched. A change of

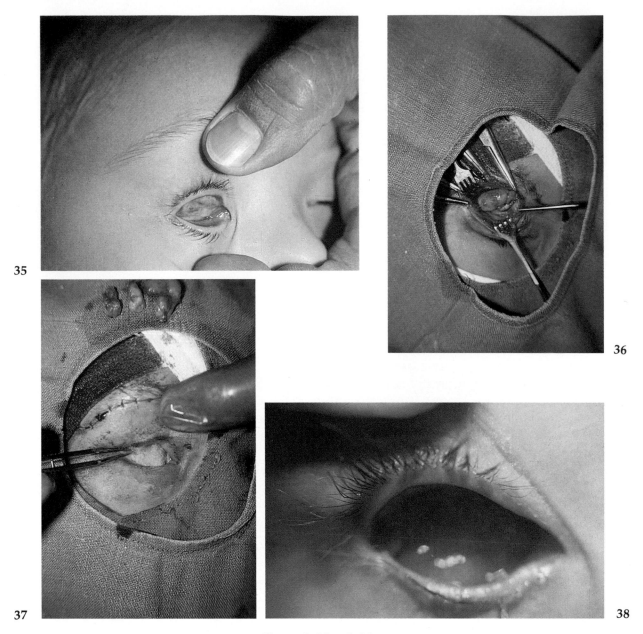

35

36

37

38

Figures 8–35 to 8–38

Figure 8–35 Contracted socket related to orbital scarring.
Figure 8–36 A central mass of scar tissue is removed.
Figure 8–37 The socket is packed with sea sponges.
Figure 8–38 Appearance following removal of sponges after four weeks.

gloves after the palpation of the socket is the routine. The socket is tightly packed with sea sponges covered with an antibiotic ointment (Fig. 8–37). A mild pressure bandage is used for 3 to 4 weeks and the dressing changed daily. Figure 8–38 shows the socket after 4 weeks of packing.

This operation was not designed for the treatment of the severely contracted socket that occurs with lye burns and radiation damage, or in some diseases such as Stevens-Johnson disease or Wegener's granulomatosis (Fig. 8–39).

SEVERELY CONTRACTED SOCKETS

These are extremely difficult orbits to rebuild and the patient must be aware before operation that the results are not always perfect. Alternatives to operation are for the patient to wear a black patch or have a prosthesis made to cover the socket and fit on a spectacle frame. These are often the better solutions. However, on occasion, a patient after being fully briefed on the possible results elects to have the socket rebuilt.

TECHNIQUE: RECONSTRUCTION OF A SEVERELY CONTRACTED SOCKET

General anesthesia is required.

The socket should be lined with buccal mucosa if possible. If this is insufficient and the patient is female, vaginal mucosa can be used. The socket can be lined with skin if mucous membrane is not available.

The lids are opened with sharp dissection (Fig. 8–40). In general, the whole central mass of scarred tissue must be removed. Muscles, Tenon's capsule, and fat are all caught up in this scar so it is usually impossible to preserve even the levator. In actuality, a partial exenteration is done, saving the lids.

If vaginal mucous membrane is to be used, a piece can easily be obtained from the vault of the vagina (Fig. 8–41), large enough to line the orbit adequately (Fig. 8–42). This does not impair the organ's primary function. The donor material should be obtained by a gynecologist, and the postoperative care of the donor site prescribed by him. If skin is to be used, it can be taken from the abdomen where the scar is less conspicuous than when the leg is the donor site. A split thickness graft approximately 2 in. wide and 6 in. long is taken with a Stryker or Padgett dermatome.

It is important to trim the graft carefully and suture it to the cut palpebral edges. The orbit is packed with sea sponges moistened with antibiotic solution, and the lids are sutured shut over a conformer (Fig. 8–43). The lids are left closed for 10 days. The sponges are carefully removed in stages—one at a time over the ensuing 2 weeks, care being taken not to disturb the graft.

Figure 8–44 shows the preoperative appearance with the eye closed by contraction of the socket. Figure 8–45 demonstrates the newly constructed socket lined with vaginal mucosa. Figure 8–46 is the appearance with the prosthesis in place.

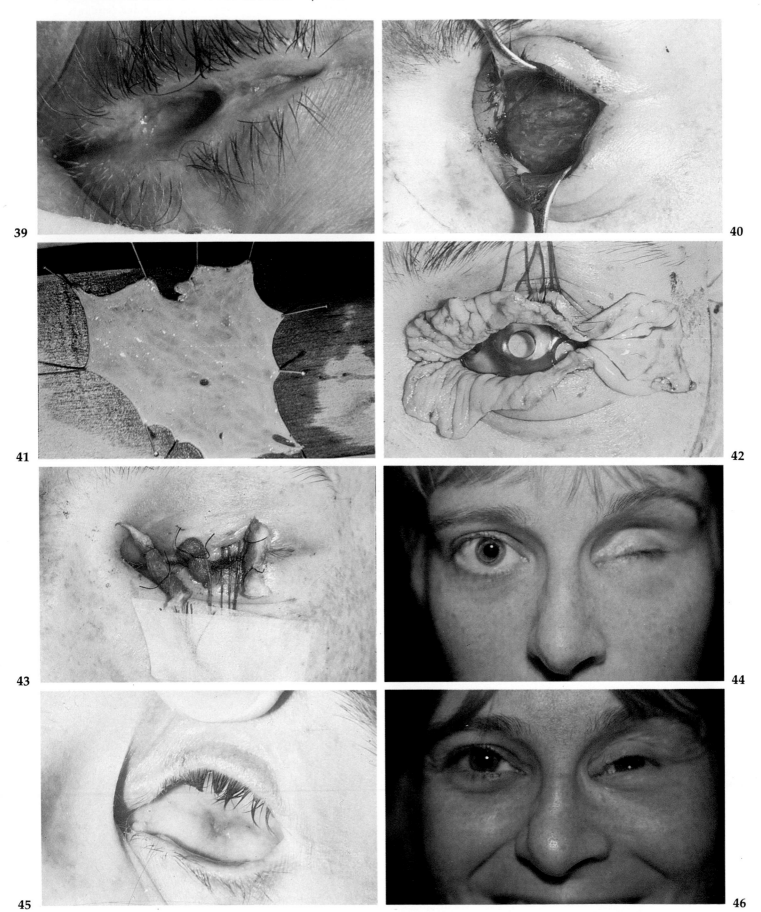

Figures 8–39 to 8–46   See opposite page for legends

CARE OF SOCKET

A socket lined with mucous membrane takes less care than one lined with skin. The mucous membrane has enough secretory glands to lubricate the prosthesis and is not disturbed by the dampness of the socket. The prosthesis need be removed only occasionally for a rinse with water.

Skin, on the other hand, is inclined to be dry and the normal desquamation must be removed daily. Frequently, leaving the prosthesis out at night permits the skin to "breathe" and helps in the normal care. A skin lotion is useful in cleaning the orbit and keeping the skin soft and pliable.

Figures 8–39 to 8–46

Figure 8–39   The socket obliterated as a result of Wegener's granulomatosis.
Figure 8–40   Sharp dissection is used to open the lids.
Figures 8–41 and 8–42   Vaginal mucous membrane is used to line the socket.
Figure 8–43   Lids are sutured over a conformer.
Figure 8–44   Preoperative, lids are scarred shut.
Figures 8–45 and 8–46   Postoperative.

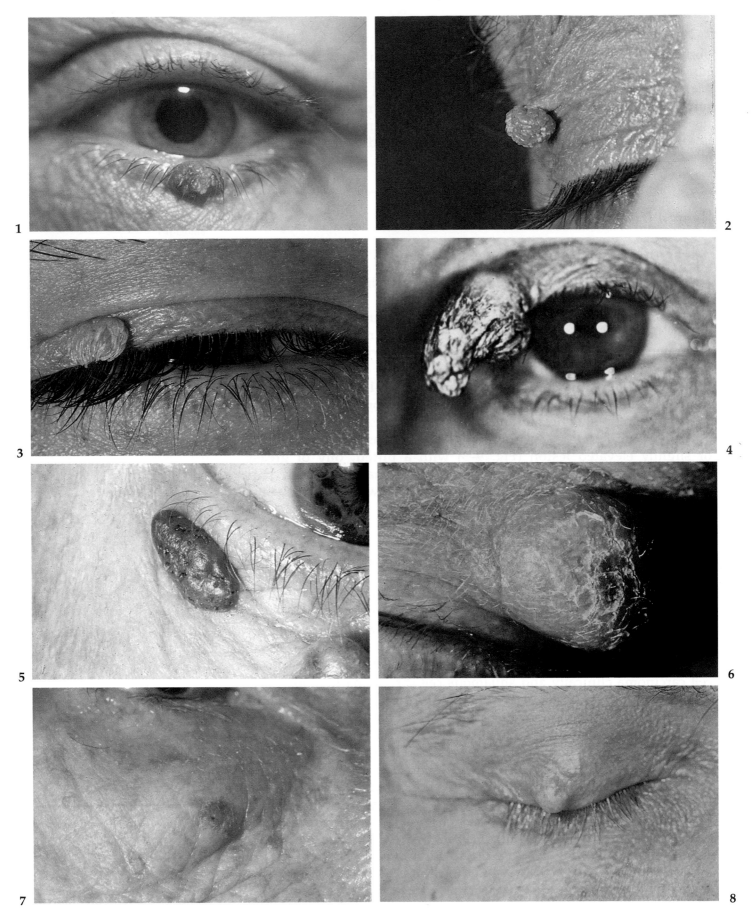

they are usually only slightly elevated, they may present as a cutaneous horn. Senile keratosis is significant because it may develop into a squamous cell carcinoma, but as a premalignant entity it is treated with simple excision.

ADNEXAL ORIGIN

Sebaceous Adenomas and Trichoepitheliomas. These are uncommon tumors with no clinically distinguishing characteristics. Trichoepitheliomas (which may arise from the cilia) usually appear at the lid margin.

Pilomatrixomas. A rare benign tumor of hair follicles, a pilomatrixoma usually occurs in young adults. It consists of a localized, encapsulated hard nodule of the lid and brow up to 3 cm in diameter that moves freely over the deep tissues but adheres to overlying skin.

CYSTIC TUMORS

Epithelial Inclusion Cysts. These cysts occur anywhere around the eyes (Fig. 9–8) but are more common near the inner and outer canthi. They result from the trapping of epithelium below the surface, possibly in a hair shaft or gland orifice. This island of epithelium continues to grow and forms a cyst with an epithelial lining that is filled with keratin debris. These cysts invariably begin with a connection to the surface, but this may not be apparent at the time of excision. It is important to remove the cyst intact, as the keratin debris is quite irritating to the surrounding tissue.

Apocrine hydrocystomas. Small, epithelium-lined cysts (Fig. 9–9) of sweat gland origin, these occur along the mucocutaneous junction or lash margin of the lids and at the inner and outer canthal areas. They are clear and transilluminate well and are usually from 1 to 5 mm in diameter but may be as large as 1 cm. They are easily excised or marsupialized.

Milia. These occur as a result of the obstruction of a pilar shaft with a subsequent build-up of keratin debris. They present as small white or yellowish round slightly elevated lesions.

Comedones. Blackheads, or comedones, are caused by occlusion of the pilosebaceous follicles and contain keratotic debris and inspissated secretion.

NEVI

Nevi are congenital lesions composed of cells of neuroectodermal origin. They occur frequently on the surface of the lid or the lid margin (Fig. 9–10), and if large, a marked thickening of the lid can result (Fig. 9–11). Nevi may have varying degrees of pigmentation

Figures 9–1 to 9–3 Papillomas.
Figure 9–4 Cutaneous horn.
Figure 9–5 Seborrheic keratosis.
Figure 9–6 Molluscum contagiosum.
Figure 9–7 Senile keratosis.

Figure 9–8 Epithelial inclusion cyst.
Figure 9–2 Courtesy of Dr. Rudolph Franklin.
Figures 9–5, 9–6 Courtesy of Dr. W. R. Green Wilmer Institute, Department of Ophthalmic Pathology.

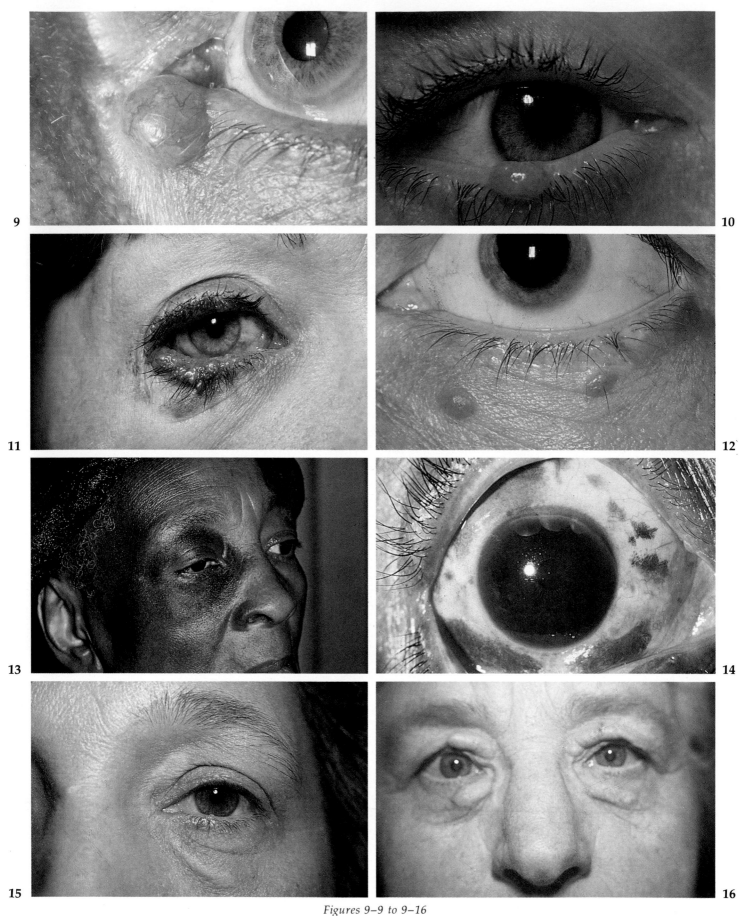

Figures 9–9 to 9–16

228

Figure 9–9 Apocrine hydrocystoma.
Figure 9–10 Marginal nevus.
Figure 9–11 Nevus involving both lids.
Figure 9–12 Dermal nevus on the right, the lesion inferiorly to the left is a basal cell carcinoma.
Figures 9–13 and 9–14 Nevus of Ota.
Figure 9–15 Xanthelasma.
Figure 9–16 Xanthomas.

or may be nonpigmented. The most common nevi are categorized by their histologic location. The dermal nevus, the common mole, is located entirely in the dermis and is rarely apparent before puberty. It may have a smooth, usually elevated, surface or may be papillomatous. The presence of hair (Fig. 9–12) on the surface of a nevus is evidence that it is the benign dermal type; a functional or compound nevus with malignant potential rarely has hair.* Junctional nevi arise in the deep layers of the surface epithelium and the underlying dermis and are potentially malignant tumors that appear as flat smooth lesions of variable pigmentation. The compound nevus contains both junctional and dermal elements. It is more common than the purely junctional nevus, may be elevated, and can undergo malignant change. The blue nevus is a slightly elevated lesion, blue-gray to black in color, that is usually present at birth or appears soon thereafter and does not change in size. The blue appearance results from the nevus cells being located deep in the dermis.

Oculodermal melanocytosis (nevus of Ota) is a unilateral condition that involves the skin about the eye, the conjunctiva, the sclera, and the uveal tract. It is a congenital condition that may be visible at birth or may become apparent in young adulthood (Figs. 9–13 and 9–14). There is an increased incidence of malignant melanomas of the uveal tract in this condition.†

Nevi may change in pigmentation during puberty or pregnancy as a result of hormonal influence. This is not a sign of tumor growth. However, in an older patient a change in size or elevation, an increase in pigmentation, or the presence of inflammation or ulceration all may be signs of malignant change, and the tumor should be treated accordingly. In the absence of evidence of malignant change, the approach to nevi is a conservative one.

Xanthelasmas

Xanthelasmas (Fig. 9–15), or xanthomas (Fig. 9–16), are benign, usually bilateral and symmetrical lesions seen in adults, most commonly in middle-aged females. In adults the cholesterol levels are usually normal. When xanthomas occur in a young patient, there is often associated hyperlipidemia. These lesions present as irregular yellow plaques in and beneath the skin of the lids, which usually begin near the inner canthus and spread temporally. Occasionally, skin grafting is necessary after excision to close large areas. It is important to remove all the yellowish tumor material to prevent recurrence.

Inflammatory Lesions

Inflammations and infections may be bacterial or viral.
Hordeola. Styes, or hordeola (Fig. 9–17), are bacterial infec-

---

*Hogan, M. J., and Zimmerman, L. E.: *Ophthalmic Pathology,* 2nd ed. W. B Saund .ers, Philadelphia, 1962.
†Yanoff, M., and Fine, B. S.: *Ocular Pathology, A Text and Atlas,* Hagerstown, Harper & Row, 1975, p. 635.

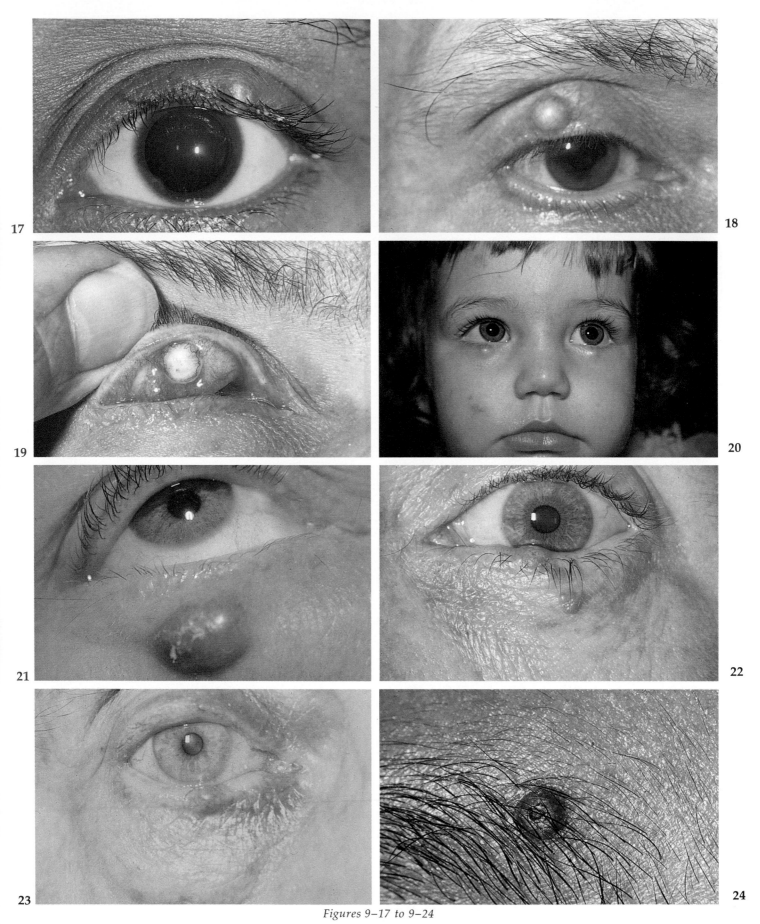

Figures 9–17 to 9–24

Figure 9–17 Hordeolum. Courtesy of Dr. David Guyton.

Figure 9–18 to 9–21 Chalazions

Figure 9–22 Chalazion of the lid margin and inferiorly a nevus of the lid.

Figure 9–23 Basal cell carcinoma of the lid margin.

Figure 9–24 Pseudoepitheliomatous hyperplasia.

tions of the meibomian glands or of the accessory glands and the lash follicles. Diagnosis is rarely difficult, and they are best treated with hot compresses, topical antibiotics, and lid hygiene. If these conservative measures do not resolve the situation satisfactorily, incision and drainage or curettage may be necessary.

Chalazions. Figures 9–18, 9–19, and 9–20 show three sites of chalazions, which arise as a result of obstruction of the opening of a meibomian gland. Inspissated lipid material causes pressure necrosis and inflammation of the gland. Subsequently there is a thickening of the tarsus and formation of a lipogranuloma. The associated inflammation often produces a pyogenic granuloma in the conjunctiva of the inner surface of the lid, which may present as a polypoid mass or anteriorly, as a soft tumor under the skin (Fig. 9–21). Occasionally it will separate from the tarsus and become movable. A chalazion has a chronic painless course unless it becomes infected, in which case it will resemble a hordeolum. Occasionally a chalazion may be difficult to distinguish from a basal cell carcinoma or nevus (Figs. 9–22 and 9–23).

Pseudoepitheliomatous Hyperplasia. This condition (Fig. 9–24) occurs in the presence of some chronic irritating factor such as a chalazion. It can occur in association with areas of chronic ulceration, foreign body, lupus vulgaris, blastomycosis infection, or basal cell carcinoma. There is a proliferation of squamous epithelium producing a tumor mass that histologically gives an appearance of a squamous cell carcinoma. Lack of invasion through the basement membrane is a key factor in the diagnosis.

Pyogenic Granulomas. These are masses of highly vascular granulation tissues that occur in response to a minor injury that has become infected (Fig. 9–25). They have a reddish color, and for this reason and their vascular nature, they may be misdiagnosed as hemangiomas.

Molluscum Contagiosum. This viral infection produces a small round elevated nodule that often has an umbilicated center from which a yellowish cheesy material can be expressed (Fig. 9–26). When the nodule is on the lid margin, virus particles and cellular debris fall into the conjunctival sac and often produce a follicular conjunctivitis and superficial keratitis. Curettage of the center of the lesion or complete excision is curative.

BENIGN NONEPITHELIAL TUMORS

HEMANGIOMAS

A hemangioma is a hamartomatous lesion that is congenital; it may involve any site. These tumors occur in several forms, and each presents differently, has a different clinical significance, and is managed in a different fashion.

Port Wine Stain. This is a telangiectatic type of hemangioma consisting of dilated and newly formed capillaries in the dermis (Fig. 9–27). It does not change in size and does not fade with aging. When present in the distribution of the first division of the fifth cranial nerve, it may have associated choroidal and cerebral heman-

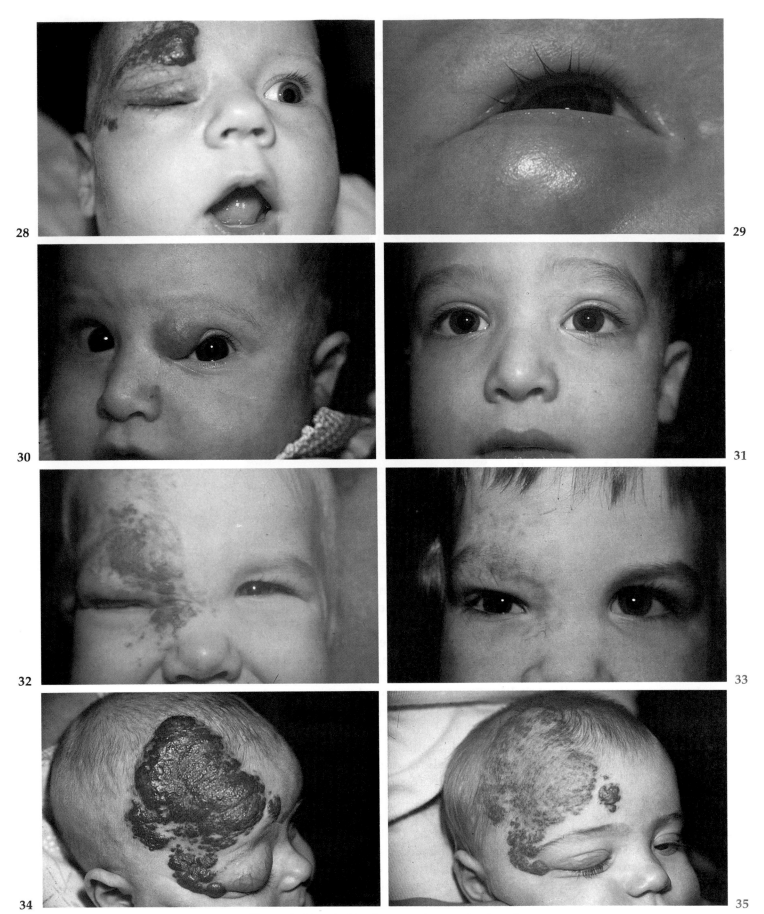

28   29

30   31

32   33

34   35

Figures 9–28 to 9–35   See opposite page for legend

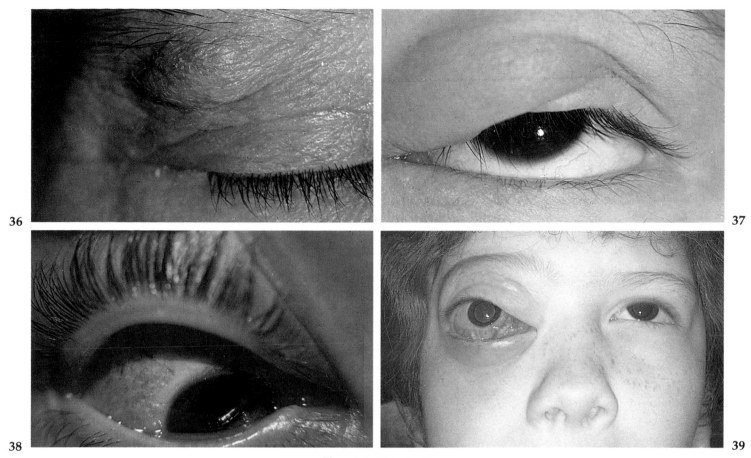

Figures 9–36 to 9–39

Figure 9–28 Diffuse capillary hemangioma.
Figure 9–29 Hemangioma of the lower lid.
Figure 9–30 Hemangioma causing astigmatism.
Figure 9–31 One year postoperative excision of hemangioma pictured in figure 9–30.
Figures 9–32 and 9–33 Pre and post treatment with small doses of irradiation.
Figures 9–34 and 9–35 Pre and post treatment with corticosteroids.
Figure 9–36 Cavernous hemangioma in an adult.
Figure 9–37 Lymphangioma of the lid.
Figure 9–38 Dilated lymphatics in the conjunctiva associated with orbital lymphangioma.
Figure 9–39 Hemorrhage into a lymphangioma can cause sudden proptosis.

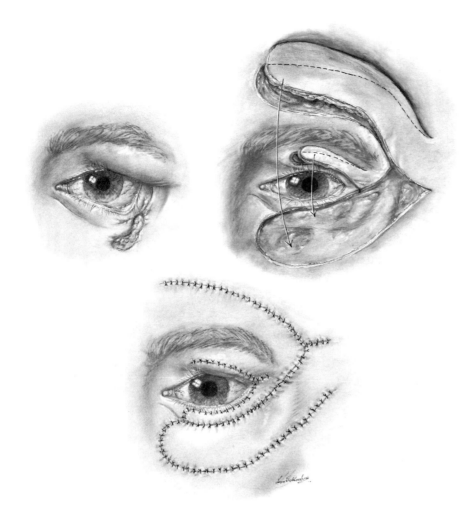

Figure 9–63

Illustration of brow and lid skin pedicle flaps used for reconstruction following the removal of a basal cell carcinoma involving the lid skin and the cheek.

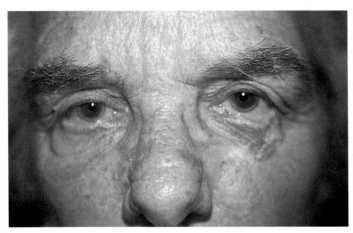

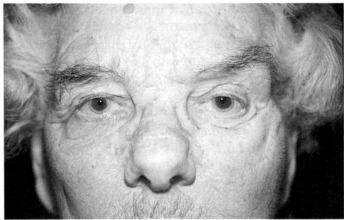

64   **65**

Figure 9–64 and Figure 9–65

Pre and postoperative views of a patient on which brow and lid pedicle flaps were used. The carcinoma extended down to the periosteum.

Figure 9–66   Basal cell carcinoma involving the skin and tarsus of the lower lid.
Figure 9–67   Dissection is started away from the lid margin.
Figures 9–68 and 9–69   The tumor is excised with removal of the least possible amount of tarsus.
Figure 9–70   Frozen sections are done on the remaining margins.
Figure 9–71   Forty percent of the tarsus was removed in this case.
Figures 9–72 and 9–73   Considerable tension would be placed on the incision therefore the lateral canthal ligament to the lower lid was cut.

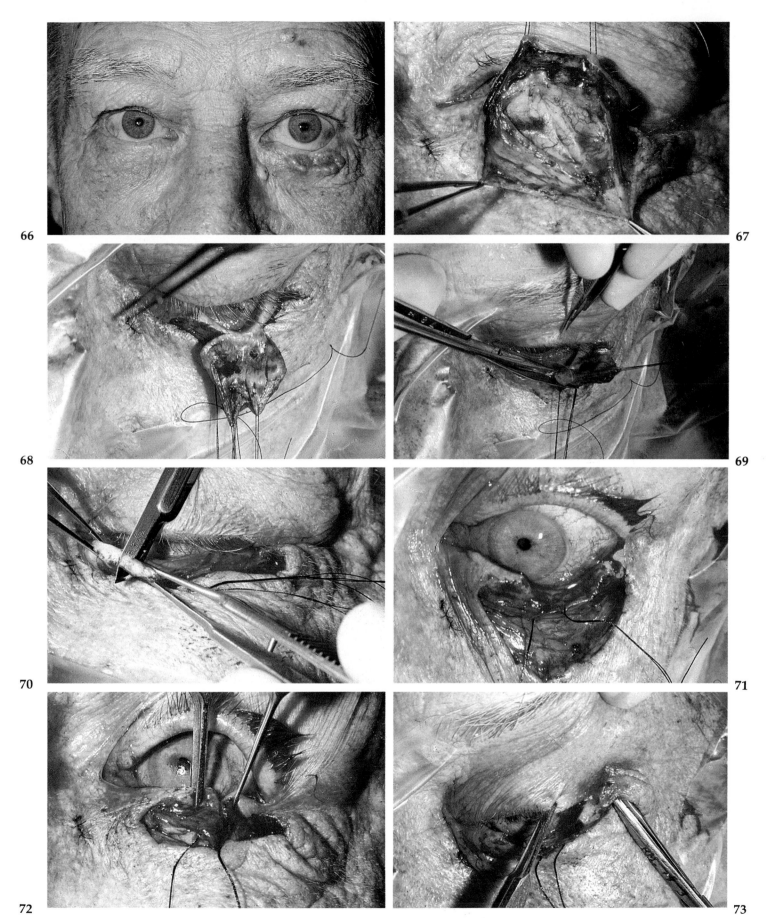

66

67

68

69

70

71

72

73

Figures 9–66 to 9–73   See opposite page for legends.

247

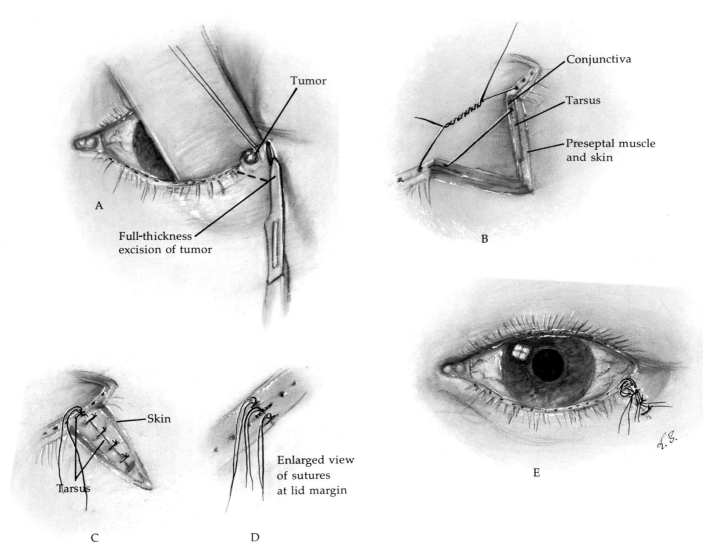

Figure 9–74 Tumors involving up to 40 per cent of lid tarsus and skin can be closed primarily. Figures 9–66 to 9–82 depict a procedure in which the skin involvement was considerably more extensive than that of the tarsus; however, the basic lid closure is carried out in the same fashion.

Figures 9–75 to 9–82

Figure 9–75   The lid margin is approximated initially.
Figures 9–76 and 9–77   The tarsus is carefully reapproximated.
Figures 9–78 and 9–79   Multiple Z-plasties provide mobilization of skin to fill the anterior portion of the defect.
Figure 9–80   The patient in figures 66 to 79, six months postoperatively.
Figure 9–81   Moderately sized basal cell carcinoma involving the right upper lid.
Figure 9–82   The patient in figure 9–81 three years after surgery. The tumor was excised, the area closed primarily and the extension of the lateral canthal ligament to the upper lid cut to allow the temporal half of the lid to slide nasally.

248

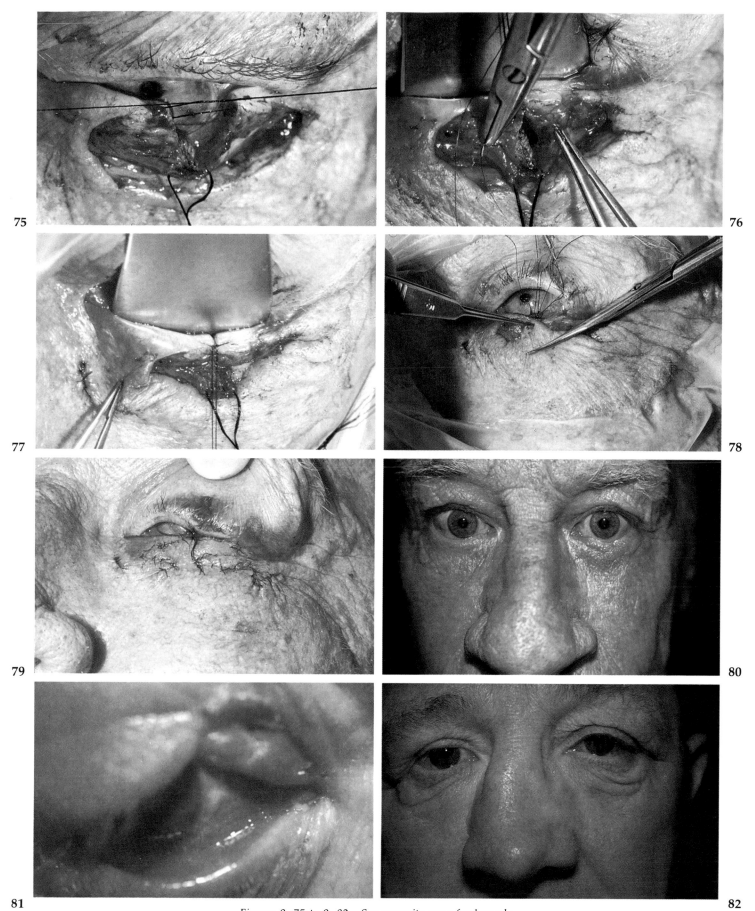

75

76

77

78

79

80

81

82

Figures 9–75 to 9–82   See opposite page for legends.

249

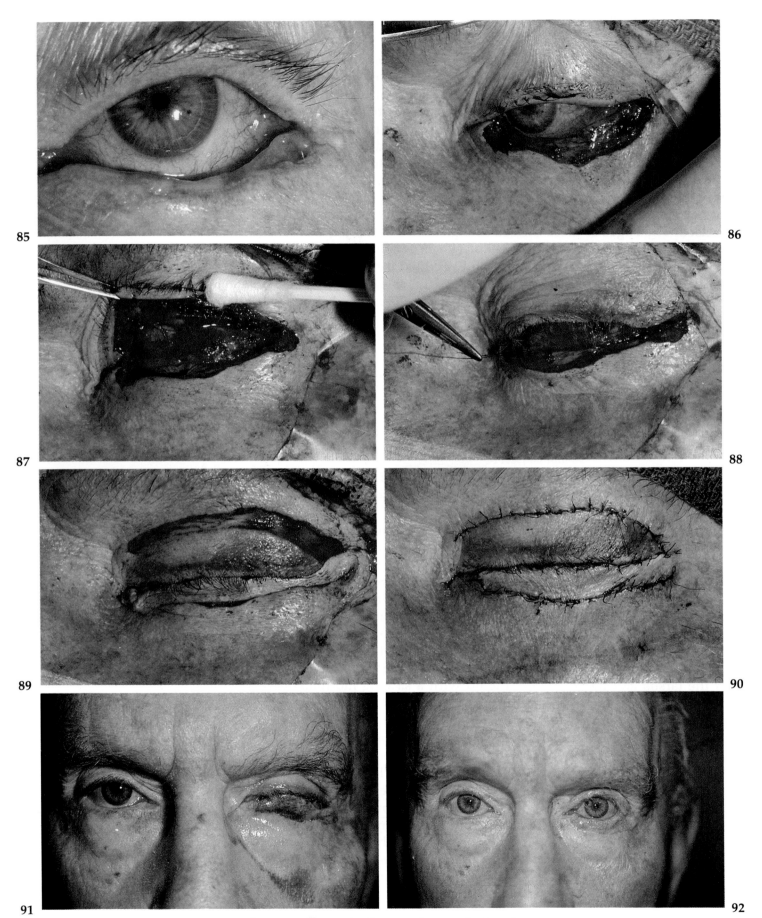

85

86

87

88

89

90

91

92

Figures 9–85 to 9–92   See opposite page for legends.

254

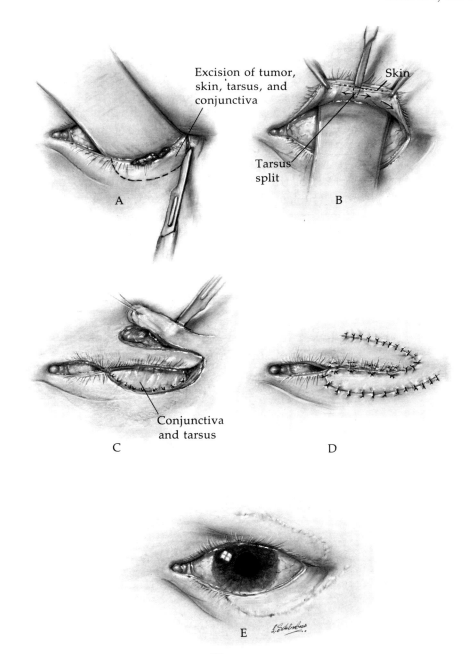

Figure 9–93

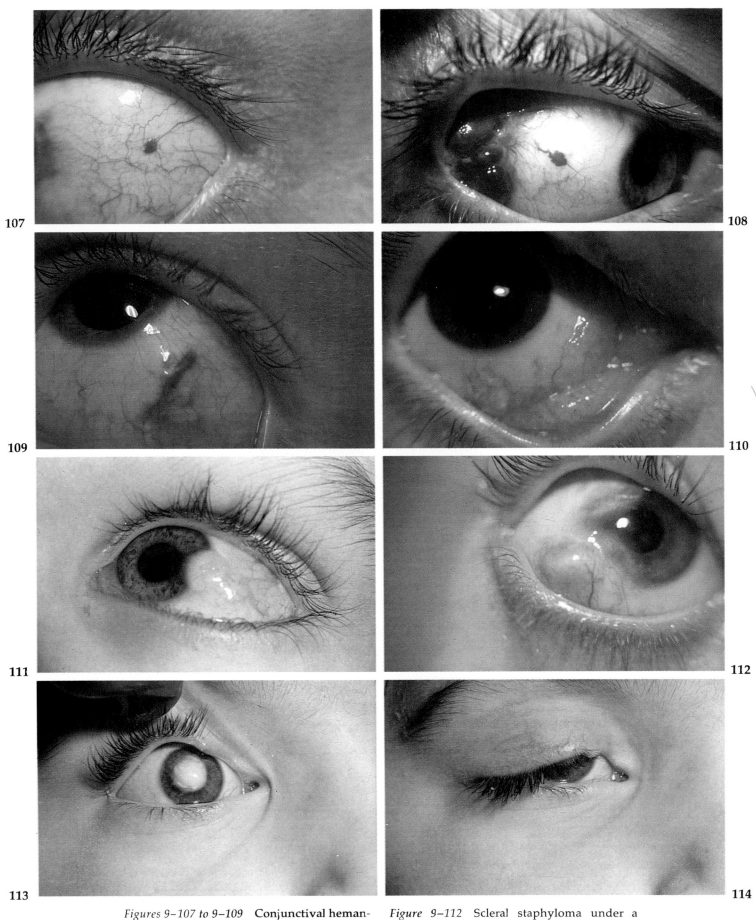

107

108

109

110

111

112

113

114

266

Figures 9–107 to 9–109 **Conjunctival hemangiomas.**
Figure 9–110 **Lymphangioma involving the conjunctiva.**
Figure 9–111 **Limbal dermoid.**

Figure 9–112 **Scleral staphyloma under a dermoid.**
Figure 9–113 **Corneal dermoid.**
Figure 9–114 **Lid abnormality associated with central dermoid** pictured in figure 9–113.

may b
dermo

Be
penetr
neal d
cornea
lamell
round
per ce
theliu
tumor
the di
for ad
Some
the co
move
sclere
under
(Fig.
serve
defec
quire
conge
moid
const

I

I
usual
upwa
the r
lial s
fat, t
that
tumo
tion;
great
orbit
and
Too
cle i
mass
be d
edge
conji

Benign Tumors

HEMANGIOMAS

Hemangiomas are occasionally found in the buibar and palpebral conjunctiva and are frequently associated with hemangiomas of the lids or orbit. A capillary hemangioma presents as a bright red discrete tumor of the conjunctiva (Fig. 9–107) that is freely movable over the sclera. The cavernous hemangioma may be firm yet compressible and is frequently lobulated (Figs. 9–108 and 9–109). The cavernous lesion is more likely to extend into the orbit, and when located nasally, the caruncle is often involved. Hemangiomas when well circumscribed are best treated by complete excision, with cauterization of the afferent and efferent vessels. Some hemangiomas extend into the orbit; a conservative approach is recommended, with removal of only the anterior portion of this benign lesion. In the past, some of these lesions were treated with beta irradiation and excellent results were obtained. However, beta irradiation has not in general been used in recent years as the potent beta radiation applicator is no longer available, and radium plaques have very low percentage of the beta rays and higher concentration of the deeper penetrating gamma rays, which are undesirable for this particular lesion.

LYMPHANGIOMAS

Lymphangiomas may appear in the conjunctiva as small to moderate-sized dilated tortuous vessels filled with clear fluid (Fig. 9–110) and may be evidence of an associated orbital lymphangioma. No treatment is indicated for these small vessels. However, if the conjunctiva becomes distended or pouting and projects through the lids, the excess can be excised and the edges of the incision closed with 8–0 absorbable suture.

DERMOIDS

Dermoids are choristomatous lesions that are either solid or cystic and derive from the inclusion of epidermal and associated connective tissue structures in abnormal locations during the closure of fetal fissures. They occasionally contain other tissues, including nerve bundles, fat, aberrant lacrimal and sweat glands, and brain. Limbal dermoids are firmly fastened to the cornea and penetrate the superficial stroma (Fig. 9–111). They are solid, are most commonly found in the lower temporal quadrant, and may appear as opaque pinkish-white firmly fixed masses as large as 8 to 10 mm. Although they usually involve the anterior one half of the corneal stroma, there may be intraocular extension or an underlying staphyloma (Fig. 9–112). The presence of a few hairs on the surface of the lesion is diagnostic. Dermoids may be bilateral and can occur as isolated structures on the cornea without any connection to the limbus. Vision can be impaired as a result of astigmatism or obscuring of the visual axis by tumor or lipid (Fig. 9–113). Dermoids

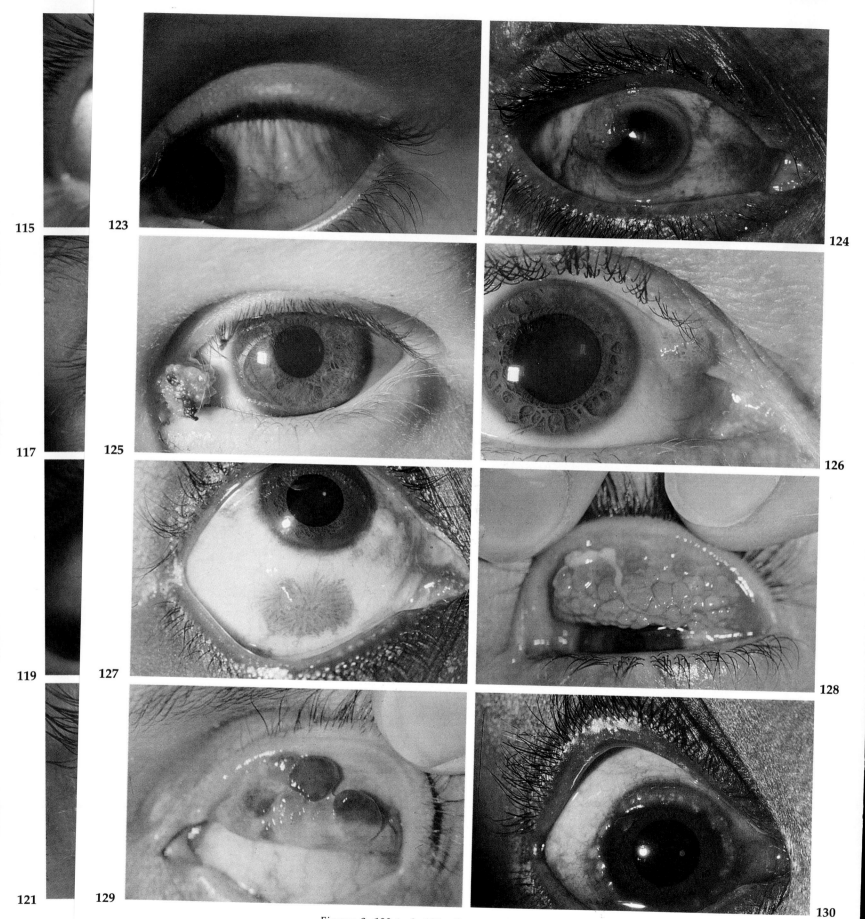

115

123

124

117

125

126

119

127

128

121

129

130

268

270

Figures 9–123 to 9–130   See opposite page for legend.

of the tumor and is separated from the tumor mass over the lateral scleral triangle without extending the dissection up and temporally into the area of the lacrimal ducts or the lacrimal glands, nor back further to the insertion of the lateral rectus muscle. The anterior portion of the tumor is cut away with cautery to control the bleeding, and the conjunctiva is closed with 8–0 buried absorbable sutures.

NEVI

The nevus is a common congenital tumor that may be single or multiple and is usually located in the interpalpebral area at or near the limbus (Figs. 9–120 and 9–121) or at the caruncle (Fig. 9–122). It may be elevated and have a slightly rough surface and variable amounts of pigmentation. This pigmenation may become more marked during pregnancy or with other changes in the hormonal balance, as with hormonal contraceptive therapy. Frequently, cystic areas are present (Fig. 9–123) in the lesion. When located at the caruncle, lanuginous hairs may grow through the tumor mass. Nevi are insensitive to irradiation, and surgical treatment is indicated for cosmetic purposes only, unless there is evidence of growth, change in pigmentation, or inflammation suggesting malignancy. Children require general anesthesia, but adults, depending on their ability to cooperate can usually be operated upon with local anesthesia. Lidocaine is infiltrated in the subconjunctival area of the tumor, providing anesthesia and facilitating excision by elevating the lesion away from the sclera. The nevus should be excised with 1 mm margins using sharp-pointed iris scissors. The elasticity of the conjunctiva aids in closure, which should be done with fine absorbable 8–0 sutures with buried knots.

PAPILLOMAS

Papillomas are moderately fast growing epithelial lesions probably of viral origin that may occur anywhere on the conjunctiva but seem to occur more frequently at the limbus (Fig. 9–124) or the caruncle (Fig. 9–125) or on the lid margin (Fig. 9–126). They may be single or multiple and occasionally are present bilaterally. In the cul-de-sac, the tumor is usually a pink, friable, pedunculated mass containing many finger-like extensions. Papillomas involving the lid margins are more compact. Trauma may cause bleeding and crusting. In such cases, bloody tears may appear and be most alarming to the patient. Limbal papillomas and those of the bulbar conjunctiva (Fig. 9–127) consist of moderately elevated masses with a flat, irregular surface. Although the origin is at the limbus, the tumor may extend over the cornea or back over the conjunctiva as

---

Figures 9–123 to 9–130

Figure 9–123 Cysts evident in limbal nevus.
Figures 9–124 to 9–127 Papillomas.
Figure 9–126 Courtesy of Dr. Rudolph Franklin.
Figure 9–128 and 9–129 Vernal conjunctivitis.
Figure 9–130 Limbal vernal conjunctivitis.

271

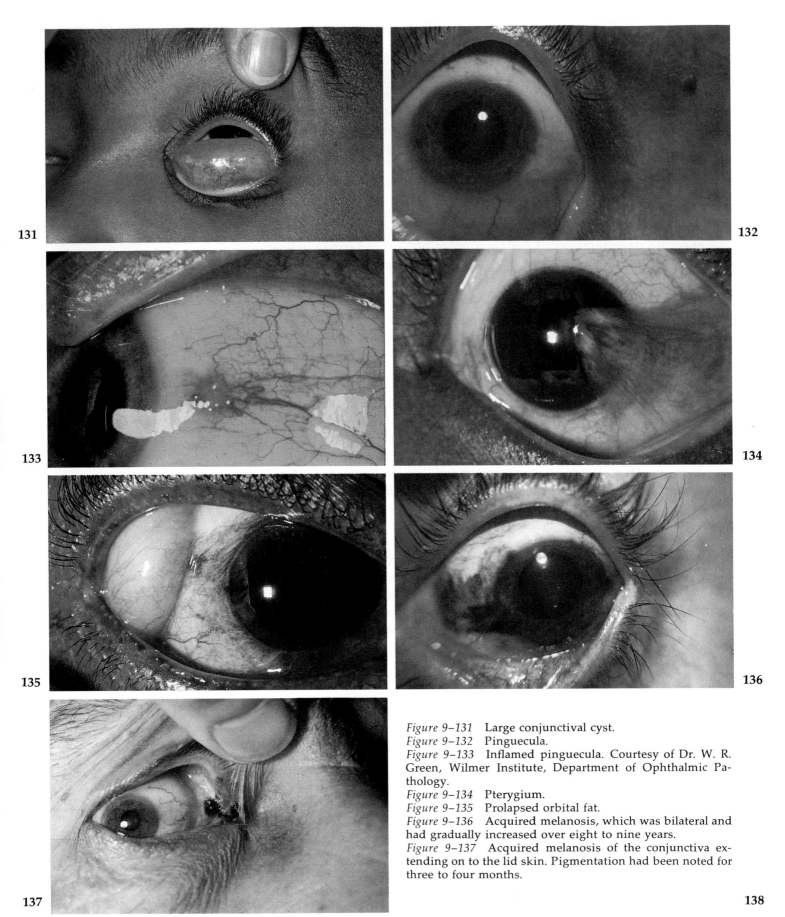

131

132

133

134

135

136

137

138

Figure 9–131   Large conjunctival cyst.
Figure 9–132   Pinguecula.
Figure 9–133   Inflamed pinguecula. Courtesy of Dr. W. R. Green, Wilmer Institute, Department of Ophthalmic Pathology.
Figure 9–134   Pterygium.
Figure 9–135   Prolapsed orbital fat.
Figure 9–136   Acquired melanosis, which was bilateral and had gradually increased over eight to nine years.
Figure 9–137   Acquired melanosis of the conjunctiva extending on to the lid skin. Pigmentation had been noted for three to four months.

Figures 9–131 to 9–137

tomy to the depth of clear cornea. Any small remaining tags of the pterygium that remain on the cornea will produce new vascularization to this point and must be removed. To do this, some surgeons use a diamond dust drill or a small dental drill to polish the corneal lamellae. The lamellar keratectomy is carried as far as the limbus and then the superficial sclera is shaved so the pterygium is removed *in toto*. All bleeding points are closed with mild cautery. The conjunctiva covering the body of the pterygium is completely excised. The edges of the conjunctival incision are slightly undermined and the conjunctiva from above and below is mobilized to close over the defect, using 8–0 absorbable suture and leaving a 3 mm bare scleral area at the limbus. Another approach to closure is rotating a flap of conjunctiva from above or below to fill the defect. This allows the suture line to fall away from the area of the original lesion, possibly lessening the likelihood of recurrence.

Postoperatively, steroid drops are used two or three times a day. In the past, beta irradiation was given over the bare sclera at the limbus at the time of operation. However, in a high percentage of these cases, a localized cataract was produced that in many instances did not appear for 6 to 8 years. For this reason, this treatment is now rarely used.

PROLAPSED ORBITAL FAT

Prolapsed orbital fat under the conjunctiva (Fig. 9–135) is usually a bilateral condition and is believed to be caused by a congenital weakness in Tenon's capsule that progresses with age.* The fat usually presents between the lateral and superior rectus muscles, but it can also be seen in the temporal scleral triangle if the prolapse is severe. The appearance is that of a soft, yellow, lobulated subconjunctival mass. The masses of fat may be cosmetically objectionable and require surgical removal, which must be undertaken with care to avoid hemorrhage or damage to the lacrimal ducts.

Following incision through conjunctiva over the fat, the lobule is clamped and the fat distal to the clamp is excised with cautery. The clamp is slowly released and any bleeders taken care of. There should be no pulling on the fat lobules for they are continuous with the orbital fat and any pulling could rupture a vessel deep in the orbit. The conjunctival incision should not be carried far superotemporally or the lacrimal ducts could be injured. The conjunctiva and Tenon's capsule are closed with absorbable sutures.

ACQUIRED MELANOSIS

Acquired melanosis of the conjunctiva is a premalignant lesion that may present as focal or diffuse flat pigmentation on the palpebral or bulbar conjunctiva (Figs. 9–136 and 9–137). Zimmerman's classification† has allowed differentiation of the benign and malignant forms

---

*Fox, S. A.: *Ophthalmic Plastic Surgery*, 5th ed. Grune & Stratton, New York, 1976, p. 462.

†Zimmerman, L. E.: Criteria for Management of Melanosis Arch. Ophthalmol. 76:307, 1966.

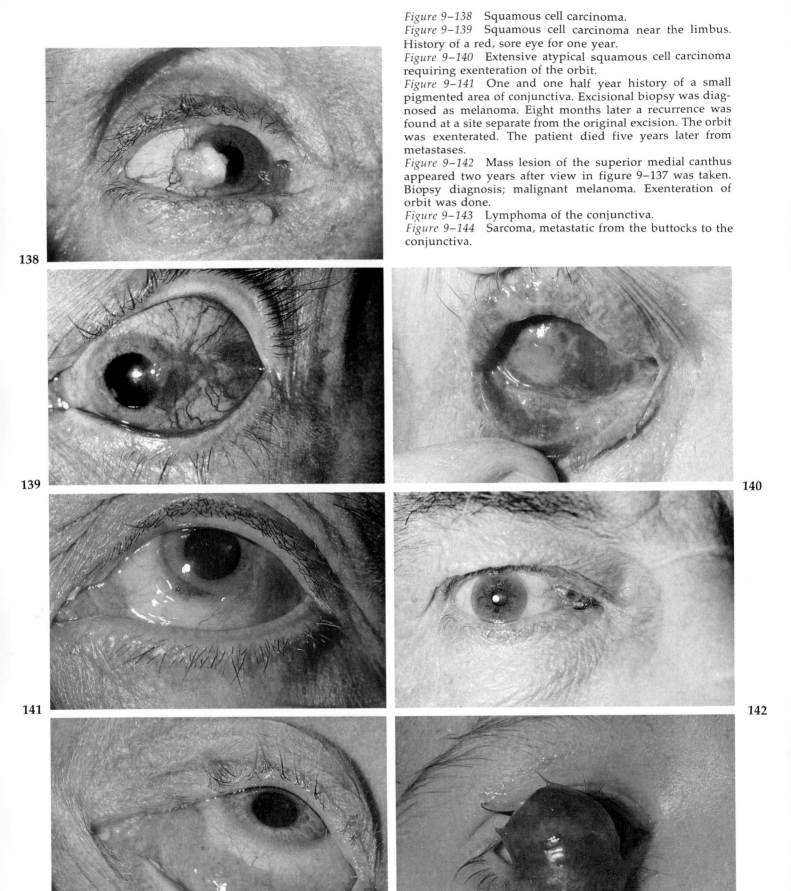

Figure 9–138 Squamous cell carcinoma.
Figure 9–139 Squamous cell carcinoma near the limbus. History of a red, sore eye for one year.
Figure 9–140 Extensive atypical squamous cell carcinoma requiring exenteration of the orbit.
Figure 9–141 One and one half year history of a small pigmented area of conjunctiva. Excisional biopsy was diagnosed as melanoma. Eight months later a recurrence was found at a site separate from the original excision. The orbit was exenterated. The patient died five years later from metastases.
Figure 9–142 Mass lesion of the superior medial canthus appeared two years after view in figure 9–137 was taken. Biopsy diagnosis; malignant melanoma. Exenteration of orbit was done.
Figure 9–143 Lymphoma of the conjunctiva.
Figure 9–144 Sarcoma, metastatic from the buttocks to the conjunctiva.

138

139

140

141

142

143

144

histologically and has given guidance in the clinical staging. In the past, radical therapy was often recommended for early stages. Benign acquired melanosis (Zimmerman: Stage 1A and 1B) is treated by biopsy, photography, and observation unless it is cosmetically significant and localized so that total excision is possible and desired by the patient. Since microscopic subclinical changes are often present, excision of a localized pigmented area does not ensure total removal. Careful follow-up and photographic documentation are important in the management of the early stages of the disease.

Malignant melanosis (malignant melanoma) (see p. 278) presents as an elevated area in a previously flat portion of melanosis. An occasional benign lesion will appear this way, but melanoma *must be ruled out by biopsy*. In addition to elevation, changes in pigmentation and signs of inflammation are evidence of malignant degeneration.

Malignant Tumors

SQUAMOUS CELL CARCINOMAS

Squamous cell carcinoma of the conjunctiva (Fig. 9–138) is a relatively rare tumor that may arise anywhere in the conjunctiva but is most common at the limbus. It usually presents as a localized, white, mildly elevated mass fed by large conjunctival vessels, but it may be diffuse and accompanied by inflammation that obscures the more typical appearance (Figs. 9–139 and 9–140). The lesion may be a carcinoma *in situ* or a noninvasive lesion or may become frankly invasive. Invasive squamous cell carcinoma of the conjunctiva fortunately seems to behave in a benign fashion, and these localized lesions do not tend to metastasize. However, deep invasion of the corneal stroma and the sclera and even intraocular invasion have been reported.*

Squamous cell carcinoma *in situ* can be managed by simple excision if the tumor has clear margins. Likewise, if the tumor is superficially invasive, excision is usually adequate, as long as adequate tumor-free margins are obtained by careful cooperation with the ophthalmic pathologist. Since this type of localized lesion does not tend to metastasize, there appears to be no need for more radical surgery.

The excision technique is similar to that for a pterygium, in which any portion that overlies the cornea is removed by limbal keratectomy while the body of the tumor is shaved from the sclera with a Gill knife. The tumor is elevated by a small sponge to control the bleeding areas as they appear. The procedure should be done under the microscope. Surrounding conjunctiva is mobilized, and the defect is completely or partially (depending on the amount of conjunctiva available) closed.

Tumor extension into the deep corneal or scleral stroma and intraocular extension require enucleation for complete removal.

*Iliff, W. J., Marback, R., and Green, W. R.: Invasive squamous cell carcinoma of the conjunctiva. Arch. Ophthalmol. 93:119, 1975.

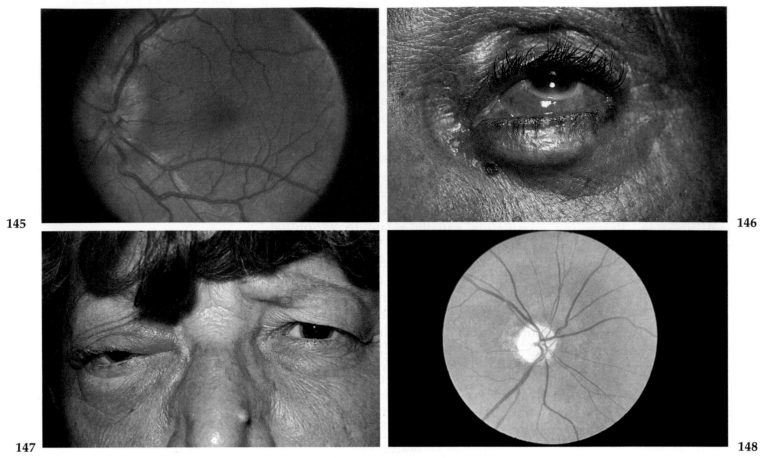

145   146

147   148

Figures 9–145 to 9–148

Figure 9–145   Retinal striae.

Figure 9–146   Pseudotumor of the orbit presenting with pain, inflammation, and lid mass.

Figure 9–147   Orbital tumor presenting with pain and inflammation. Pathology revealed metastatic breast carcinoma. (Courtesy of Dr. Neil Miller.)

Figure 9–148   Optic atrophy secondary to arachnoid cyst of the optic nerve.

of the globe can induce astigmatism. Optic disc edema or atrophy in the presence of proptosis is strong evidence for the presence of a posterior orbital tumor with involvement of the optic nerve or its blood supply. (Thyroid disease can also cause disc edema associated with exophthalmos and must be considered.) Visual field defects may be present in the absence of decreased central acuity and should be tested for in any patient suspected of having an orbital tumor. If there is venous compression, retinal vein engorgement and retinal hemorrhage may result.

Diplopia may result from invasion of an extraocular muscle or ocular motor nerve or from pressure on one of these structures by a tumor. In addition, the bulk of a mass lesion can cause diplopia by mechanically interfering with the position or motion of the globe. Strabismus without diplopia can also be a manifestation of orbital tumor, particularly if the vision in one eye is poor.

Rapidly enlarging tumors, those which invade bone or nerves, and those associated with inflammation cause pain and tenderness. Malignant mixed tumor of the lacrimal gland may cause pain by involvement of periosteum and bone. Perineural extension of adenoid cystic carcinoma of the lacrimal gland is frequently associated with pain. Inflammatory pseudotumor of the orbit can be associated with pain.

The presence of orbital inflammation (erythema, edema, tenderness) suggests infection, which most commonly originates in the paranasal sinuses. However, it should be remembered that a sinus infection may be secondary to obstruction of sinus drainage by a neoplasm. Inflammation in the absence of infection may be related to orbital pseudotumor (Fig. 9–146), thyroid disease, or other benign orbital processes. Occasionally, however, inflammatory changes may occur in or around a malignancy (Fig. 9–147).

Palpation of the orbit suggests the degree of encapsulation or the degree of fixation of a mass to surrounding structures. Dermoids, hemangiomas, and benign tumors of the lacrimal gland may feel quite discrete and be freely movable. Thyroid disease, pseudotumors, lymphomas, and secondary carcinomas usually diffusely involve the orbit, producing fixation of many orbital structures. Hemangiomas, lymphangiomas, lymphomas, and lipomas tend to be soft and compressible, permitting the eye to be retropulsed; most malignant tumors, pseudotumors, and thyroid disease tend to produce a firm, noncompressible orbit.

AGE

In children, congenital benign tumors, dermoid cysts, hemangiomas, lymphangiomas, neurofibromas, and pseudotumors are more common than malignant tumors. Rhabdomyosarcoma, the most common primary malignant tumor of the orbit, is virtually confined to the first decade of life, although an occasional well documented case has been seen in an elderly person. Gliomas of the optic nerve are in general confined to the pediatric or adolescent age group. In adults, although late-appearing congenital lesions such as hemangiomas and dermoids do occur, thyroid disease, inflammatory pseudotumor, lymphoma, and secondary tumors (metastatic or extending from contiguous structures) are more common.

SEX

The patient's sex gives little diagnostic help, except in cases of metastatic tumors from the breast, ovaries, testis, or prostate.

GROWTH

Benign lesions, particularly congenital ones, in general enlarge slowly. The exceptions are pseudotumors, which may have a very rapid course, and hemorrhage into a hemangioma or lymphangioma, which may produce an apparently precipitous growth; conversely, lacrimal gland tumors and secondary carcinomas from the lids or sinuses may enlarge quite slowly. Rapid growth is a most important aspect of rhabdomyosarcoma.

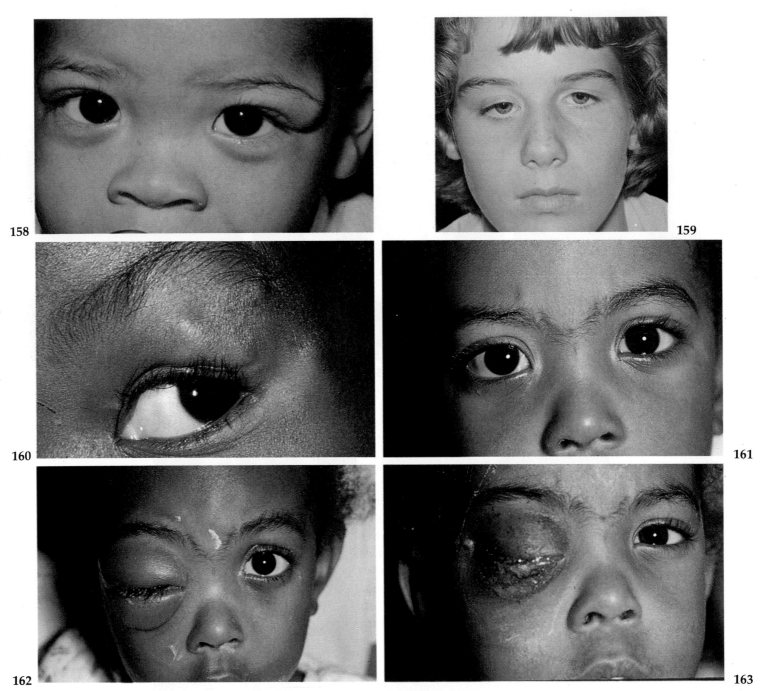

Figures 9–158 to 9–163

Figure 9–158 Supratemporal dermoid.
Figure 9–159 Deep orbital dermoid.
Figure 9–160 Multiple lid masses caused by ruptured dermoid.
Figure 9–161 Patient presented with a right orbital dermoid cyst.
Figure 9–162 The cyst ruptured at the time of surgery. Immediately postoperatively there was severe inflammation with decrease in vision to bare LP, ptosis, and sloughing of the skin.
Figure 9–163 Three weeks postoperatively. Vision has remained +− light perception.

Orbital ultrasound, though often more difficult to interpret than ocular ultrasound, can be helpful when interpreted by a person experienced in its use. Changes in orbital acoustic pattern may be subtle and a comparative sonogram of the fellow eye is needed.

The greatest advance in radiologic diagnosis of the orbit is computerized axial tomography, first developed by the E.M.I. Corporation (CT scan, CAT scan, EMI scan). The CT scan is valuable in determining the location, size, and possible type of an orbital mass (Figs. 9–154 and 9–155). With computer techniques, x-rays can be used to differentiate tissues of similar radiographic density, making possible the distinct visualization of soft tissue structures. Orbital fat provides a background of lower radiodensity, assisting in the visualization of orbital masses. Contrast studies can be done in conjunction with computerized tomography to determine if the tumor is highly vascular, as indicated by its "lighting up" on the scan. The usefulness of the CT scan is affected, as is any test, by the experience and abilities of those administering the test and interpreting the results. We found initially that the major problem in diagnosis was the misinterpretation of enlarged muscles of thyroid disease (Figs. 9–156 and 9–157) and occasionally of pseudotumor as discrete orbital masses. Improved techniques and experience have all but eliminated these causes of misdiagnosis.

Primary Orbital Tumors

DERMOID CYSTS

Dermoid cysts are slow-growing, benign tumors that occur as a result of inclusion of epithelial structures at the site of closure of a fetal fissure. They tend to be supratemporal in the orbit (Fig. 9–158) or lid but can occur deep in the orbit (Fig. 9–159). They may adhere to bone and may extend intracranially (making preoperative x-ray examination important, even for suspected brow dermoid). About 6 per cent are evident before 1 year of age, 50 per cent between 1 and 5 years of age, 8 to 10 per cent in the 6 to 10 and 11 to 15 age groups, and the remainder in adults.* Dermoids may be intermittently inflamed, presumably secondary to occasional rupture (Fig. 9–160), which occurs either spontaneously or as a result of trauma. The mass is discrete and encapsulated and may be round, oval, or lobulated. Dermoid cysts are not radiosensitive. Keeping the cysts intact during removal is essential, for the contents (keratin debris) are extremely irritating if spilled into the orbit and can cause a severe reaction (Fig. 9–161 to 9–163). If this does occur, copious irrigation and postoperative systemic steroid therapy can minimize the inflammation.

---

*Iliff, W. J., and Green, W. R.: Data presented at Wilmer Residents Association Meeting, 1975; Iliff, W. J., and Green, W. R.: Orbital tumors in children. *In* Jakobiec, F. A. (ed.): *Ocular and Adnexal Tumors.* Aesculapius Publishing Company, Birmingham, Alabama, 1978.

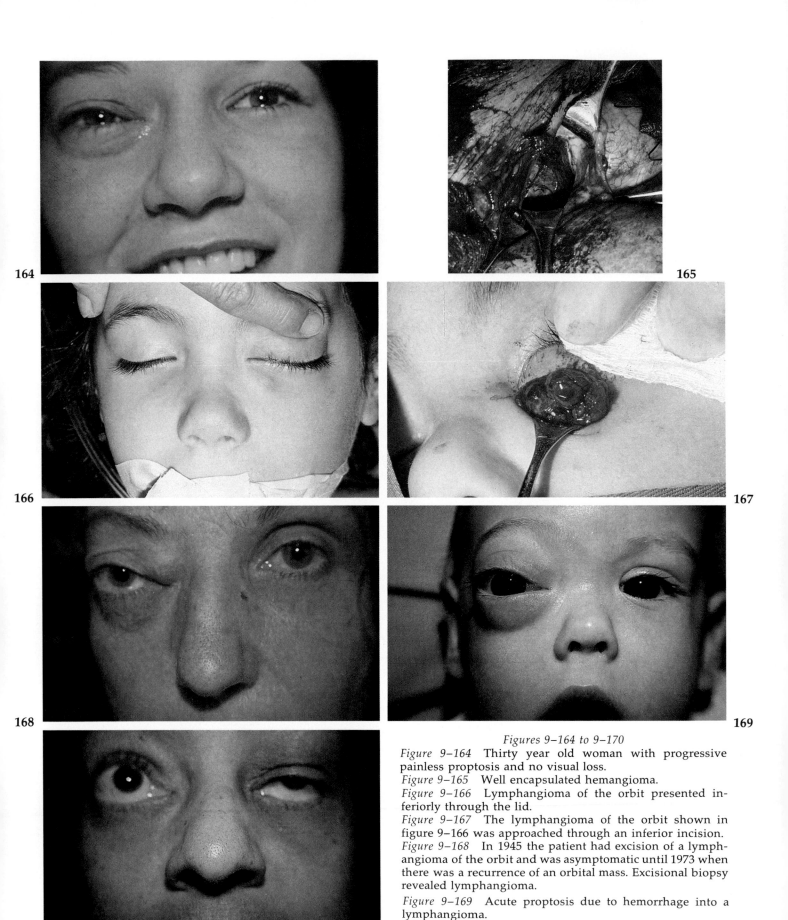

164

165

166

167

168

169

170

288

Figures 9–164 to 9–170

Figure 9–164 Thirty year old woman with progressive painless proptosis and no visual loss.

Figure 9–165 Well encapsulated hemangioma.

Figure 9–166 Lymphangioma of the orbit presented inferiorly through the lid.

Figure 9–167 The lymphangioma of the orbit shown in figure 9–166 was approached through an inferior incision.

Figure 9–168 In 1945 the patient had excision of a lymphangioma of the orbit and was asymptomatic until 1973 when there was a recurrence of an orbital mass. Excisional biopsy revealed lymphangioma.

Figure 9–169 Acute proptosis due to hemorrhage into a lymphangioma.

Figure 9–170 Left orbital pseudotumor, in this case accompanied by visual loss, ptosis and ocular muscle imbalance.

HEMANGIOMAS

Hemangiomas can occur anywhere in the orbit. In children, the presentation is usually anterior in the orbit and may involve the lids.* Management of these has been discussed under Lid Tumors, at the beginning of this chapter. Occasionally hemangiomas of the orbit may regress spontaneously as do those of the lid. Though considered congenital lesions, hemangiomas may not be symptomatic until adult life (Fig. 9–164). In this circumstance, they are characteristically discrete, oval or round, slow-growing benign tumors. They are usually well encapsulated and can be removed intact (Fig. 9–165), even if lying adjacent to the optic nerve.

LYMPHANGIOMAS

Lymphangiomas are congenital benign tumors that are usually seen in children (Figs. 9–166 and 9–167) but can present in older patients (Fig. 9–168). Dilated lymphatic channels in the conjunctiva are diagnostic of a deeper orbital lymphangioma. The deep tumor may remain undetected until hemorrhage into a lymph space causes a sudden increase in its size (Fig. 9–169). This can be severe enough that emergency decompression must be done to avoid damage to the eye. Lymphangiomas of the orbit, like those of the lid, may enlarge in the presence of an upper respiratory infection. These tumors are difficult to excise in their entirety because they do not have a capsule and considerable hemorrhage accompanies attempted excision. Drainage of hematomas and repeated partial excisions constitute the proper course of treatment. The lesions are slow growing and usually show little or no change after the patient becomes an adult.

PSEUDOTUMORS

Pseudotumors are difficult to differentiate clinically from a true neoplasm. They can occur anywhere in the orbit, are usually accompanied by pain, and can cause visual loss and a muscle imbalance (Fig. 9–170). They can be discrete or multilobulated. There may be a period of rapid enlargement (over several weeks). Treatment with systemic steroids may cause considerable decrease in the size of the tumor, but this may be misleading since an orbital mass due to malignancy also may decrease in size as a result of decrease in associated inflammation. A positive diagnosis should be made by biopsy.

---

*Iliff, W. J., and Green, W. R.: Orbital tumors in children. *In* Jakobiec, F. A. (ed.): *Ocular and Adnexal Tumors.* Aesculapius Publishing Company, Birmingham, Alabama, 1978.

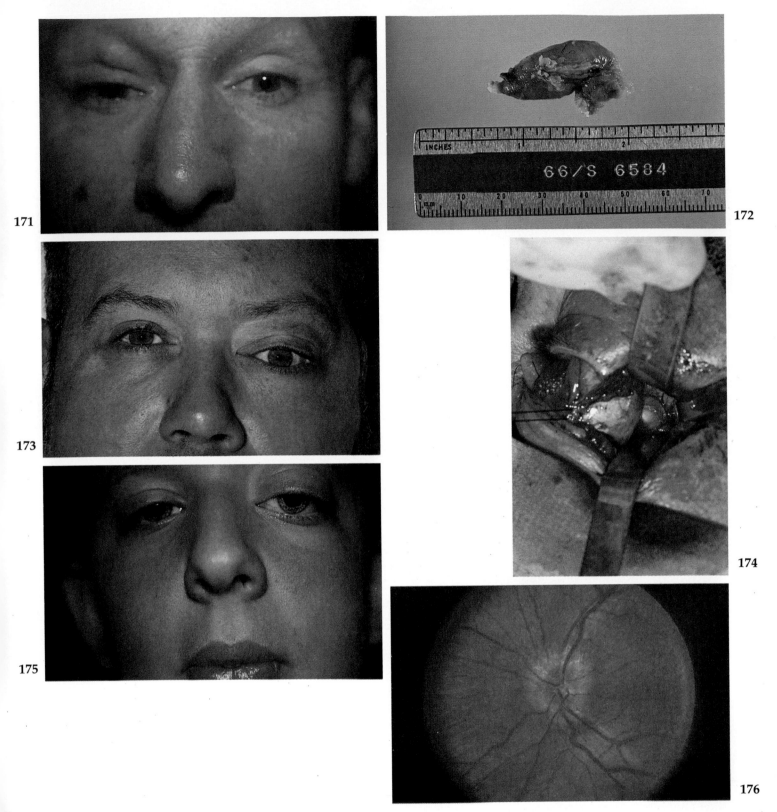

Figures 9–171 to 9–176

Figure 9–171 Neurilemmoma of frontal nerve, associated with pain and palpable mass.

Figure 9–172 Neurilemmoma excised from patient pictured in Figure 9–171.

Figure 9–173 Extensive neurofibroma of the left orbit. Patient has 20/20 vision and no diplopia.

Figure 9–174 Arachnoid cyst.

Figure 9–175 Left proptosis due to glioma of the optic nerve.

Figure 9–176 Disc edema associated with gradual decrease in vision secondary to optic nerve glioma.

NEUROFIBROMAS

Neurofibromas may be isolated lesions involving one or more nerves in the orbit or may be massive with a diffuse involvement of the orbit and lids. As a component of von Recklinghausen's disease, they occur in conjunction with neurofibromata elsewhere in the body and can be associated with optic nerve gliomas, central nervous system gliomas, and meningiomas. Café au lait spots of the skin often are a clue to the diagnosis. Numerous ocular and orbital lesions may be present, including pulsatile exophthalmos caused by a defect of the sphenoid bone with brain herniation, and iris nodules and nevi or infiltrations of the anterior chamber angle with neurofibromata causing secondary glaucoma. Isolated tumors of the orbit can be completely excised (Figs. 9–171 and 9–172), but diffuse lesions are managed best by repeated small excisions to avoid or minimize damage to uninvolved orbital structures. Complete excision is usually impossible in these cases (Fig. 9–173), and as the tumor slowly recurs, orbital decompression or even exenteration may be necessary.

LIPOMAS

Lipomas are uncommon benign orbital tumors seen in adults. They are soft and compressible and are usually located in the anterior portion of the orbit. Excision is for diagnosis and cosmetic improvement.

ARACHNOID CYSTS

Arachnoid cysts occur in adults and present a diagnostic problem that may be resolved with improved computerized tomography techniques. Progressive visual loss and bizarre visual field changes may be accompanied only by optic atrophy and no other sign or symptom. All auxiliary tests may be completely negative; the presence of a mass may be detected only by computerized tomography. The diagnosis is usually made at operation (Fig. 9–174). Marsupialization of the cyst wall stops the progressive visual loss, but there may be no improvement in vision postoperatively.

GLIOMAS

Gliomas of the optic nerve are usually noted in childhood (Fig. 9–175). Progress of the lesion is extremely slow, with gradual loss of vision due to optic nerve atrophy and gradually increasing unilateral proptosis. Retinal striae, disc edema (Fig. 9–176), and rarely, extension into the globe can occur. The tumors are believed to be benign hamartomatous lesions that are not particularly radiosensitive, and some physicians feel that surgery should be undertaken only to control progressive proptosis.* Miller, W. J. Iliff, and Green† feel

---

*Hoyt, W. F., and Baghdassarian, S. A.: Optic glioma of childhood. Natural history and rationale for conservative management. Brit. J. Ophthal. 53:793, 1969.

†Miller, N. R., Iliff, W. J., and Green, W. R.: Evaluation and management of gliomas of the anterior visual pathways. Brain 97:743, 1974.

that biopsy should be done to rule out the possibility of more serious lesions, such as meningiomas, or treatable lesions, such as arachnoid cysts of the optic nerve. Although they agree that management of optic nerve gliomas is still controversial and that it is difficult to make the decision to biopsy the optic nerve, particularly if vision is good, Miller, Iliff, and Green suggest that excision of the tumor is not necessary if adequate biopsy to confirm diagnosis can be done, proptosis is not severe, and vision remains, since gliomas of the nerve (as differentiated from malignant lesions) are not life-threatening tumors. It must be noted that the arachnoidal proliferation that may surround a glioma can be confused with that of a meningioma if only a superficial biopsy is taken. Therefore, a deep biopsy (with the certainty of visual field defect) is necessary. However, C. E. Iliff and Walsh* feel that the entire lesion should be removed at the time of diagnosis to forestall future problems (surgery for increasing proptosis) and to put the patient's mind at rest that the tumor has been totally removed (Figs. 9–177 and 9–178). It should be pointed out however, that in most cases in which the entire nerve and blood supply to the globe has been removed, the eye does not do well and damage to ocular muscles may result from the surgery, leading to a worse cosmetic situation.

RHABDOMYOSARCOMA

Rhabdomyosarcoma is the most common malignant tumor in the orbit in children (Fig. 9–179). They occur, although rarely, in adults (Fig. 9–180). Presentation (which usually is in the orbit, but may be in the lid or conjunctiva) is characterized by precipitous growth. The first sign of the condition may be an apparently trivial swelling of the lids. The time between onset and diagnosis is often short because the tumor grows rapidly (usually over a few weeks) (Fig. 9–181). Management consists of a combination of surgery, chemotherapy, and irradiation. If no metastases are detected, exenteration should be done (Figs. 9–182 to 9–184). The orbit should not be filled with any material because detection of a recurrence would be hindered, but it should be lined with a split-thickness skin graft. Chemotherapy should be started at the time of surgery and continued postoperatively.

If extension out of the orbit or metastases are known preoperatively, treatment consists only of irradiation and chemotherapy. Orbital recurrence and later metastases are treated with irradiation and chemotherapy (Fig. 9–185).

*Walsh, F. B. personal communication.

Figures 9–177 and 9–178   Optic nerve glioma.

Figure 9–179   Rhabdomyosarcoma. Patient died six weeks postoperatively.

Figure 9–180   Seventy-two year old patient with rhabdomyosarcoma; refused exenteration and received irradiation treatment. Died six months following diagnosis.

Figure 9–181   Patient presented with a small mass of the lid following an upper respiratory infection. Within two weeks the lesion had increased to this size.

Figure 9–182   One month old with an embryonal rhabdomyosarcoma.

Figure 9–183   Patient shown in figure 9–182 seven years post exenteration.

Figure 9–184   The patient pictured in 9–183 wearing prosthesis.

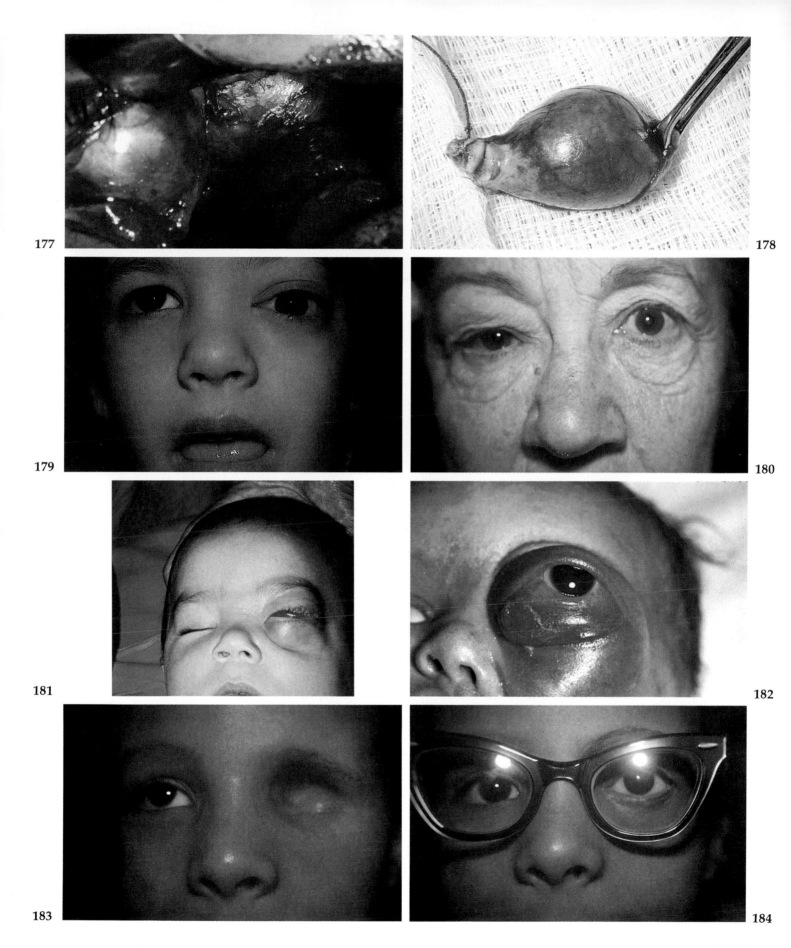

Figures 9–177 to 9–184.   See opposite page for legend.

293

MENINGIOMAS

Meningiomas of the orbit occur more commonly in adults (Fig. 9–186) but can be seen in children (Fig. 9–187). There is a definite association with neurofibromatosis; other tumors may also occur in the same patient. Depending on its location, a tumor may produce loss of vision, bizarre field defects and muscle imbalance, exophthalmos, retinal striae, or disc edema (Fig. 9–188). They are not sensitive to irradiation, and although they may seem to be circumscribed (Figs. 9–189 and 9–190), they are invasive and excision short of exenteration may result in a recurrence (Fig. 9–191). The experience of C. E. Iliff and Frank B. Walsh has been most discouraging in spite of these drastic measures, because of the associated multiple intracranial lesions that occur in many cases.

LYMPHOMAS

Lymphoma, confined to the orbit can occur, and after excisional biopsy the prognosis is quite good and the recurrence rate low. In general, however, when a lymphoma of the orbit is present, it is a manifestation of systemic involvement (Fig. 9–192). The onset of proptosis or development of a palpable mass is usually insidious and painless. The most commonly affected age group is 30 to 40 year olds, but lymphomatous diseases may occur at any age. Total excision is not possible, and a biopsy is taken for diagnosis only. Following this, the patient should be started on chemotherapy or irradiation or both, according to the type of tumor.

LACRIMAL GLAND TUMORS

Fifty per cent of lacrimal gland tumors are lymphomatous or pseudotumors (Fig. 9–193); the remainder are of epithelial origin.*

BENIGN MIXED TUMORS

Benign mixed tumors are the most common lacrimal gland tumors (Figs. 9–194 and 9–195). They usually occur in adults who are between 30 and 50 years old, but they have been reported in children. The malignant forms of mixed tumors tend to occur in older patients. The tumor is usually hard, nodular, and slightly mobile, lying just beneath the orbital rim in the lacrimal area. There usually is a slowly progressing downward and nasal proptosis.

The exact surgical management of lacrimal tumors depends on the nature and extent of the lesion found at exploration, the evidence of bone involvement, and the histology of the lesion. Benign mixed tumors should be excised completely, great care being taken to avoid rupturing the pseudocapsule. If periosteum is adherent, it should be removed without being separated from the tumor. Wide excision is important to prevent recurrences, as strands of tumor extend through the pseudocapsule. Exenteration may be required for a recurrent benign mixed tumor.

*Hogan, M. J., and Zimmerman, L. E.: *Ophthalmic Pathology*, 2nd ed. W. B. Saunders Co., Philadelphia, 1963.

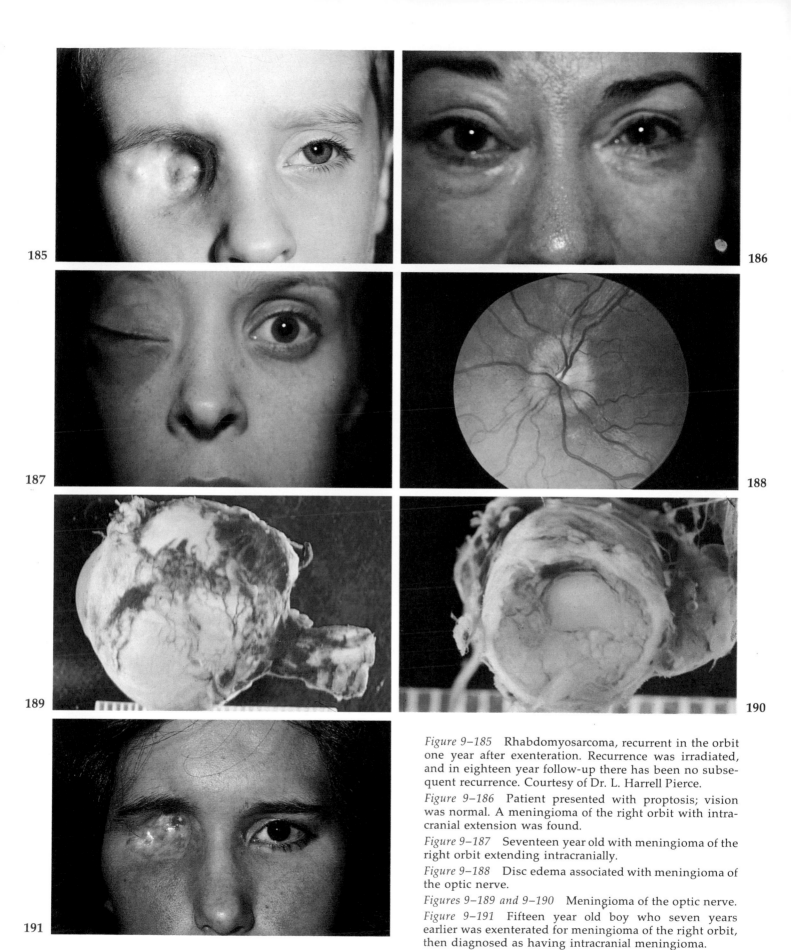

185

186

187

188

189

190

191

Figure 9–185 Rhabdomyosarcoma, recurrent in the orbit one year after exenteration. Recurrence was irradiated, and in eighteen year follow-up there has been no subsequent recurrence. Courtesy of Dr. L. Harrell Pierce.

Figure 9–186 Patient presented with proptosis; vision was normal. A meningioma of the right orbit with intracranial extension was found.

Figure 9–187 Seventeen year old with meningioma of the right orbit extending intracranially.

Figure 9–188 Disc edema associated with meningioma of the optic nerve.

Figures 9–189 and 9–190 Meningioma of the optic nerve.

Figure 9–191 Fifteen year old boy who seven years earlier was exenterated for meningioma of the right orbit, then diagnosed as having intracranial meningioma.

ADENOID CYSTIC CARCINOMA

Adenoid cystic carcinoma is the most common malignant epithelial tumor of the lacrimal gland; it occurs in adults. The tumor is very invasive, with a strong tendency to infiltrate between tissue planes and along nerves and blood vessels. Bone invasion is common; the prognosis is poor due to recurrences, intracranial spread, and metastases.

The proper treatment for adenoid cystic carcinoma of the lacrimal gland is controversial. Since it is a highly malignant tumor, exenteration and subsequent radiotherapy are advocated. Combined large resections of orbit and skull, as suggested by Wright,* have not as yet been proved to be statistically better in prolonging life than wide local tumor excision as recommended by Henderson†. Removal of underlying bone in an effort to assure complete tumor removal presents two problems. (1) The surgeon cannot be sure of the extent of the involvement from the appearance of the bone at the time of surgery, and (2) the expertise of the pathologist cannot be employed to monitor the extent of bone removal since decalcification for bone study takes several days. Thus, the procedure necessary to establish reasonable certainty that all involved bone is removed is so mutilating that its justification can be questioned, particularly since the mortality rate may not be changed.

Secondary Orbital Tumors

BENIGN SECONDARY ORBITAL TUMORS

Benign, nonmalignant secondary tumors are rare. Secondary tumors of the orbit in adults may occur as an extension from contiguous structures, including sinuses, lids, and globe.

Infections secondary to sinus disease and from distant areas occur in both children and adults (Figs. 9–196 and 9–197) and are treated with appropriate antibiotics, decongestants, and incision and drainage as needed.

OSTEOMA

Osteomas of the orbit originate primarily in the paranasal sinuses of adults and involve the orbit secondarily. Most are extremely hard and compact; they are generally sessile but may be pedunculated. Clinically, the tumors are very slow growing and may be accompanied by palpebral edema, chemosis, and headache. Optic atrophy from compression of the nerve may occur if the tumor lies near the orbital apex. The most common origin is the frontal sinus, followed by the ethmoid, the maxillary antrum, and the sphenoid. Sinusitis, nasolacrimal obstruction, and cranial nerve damage can occur. Direction of proptosis depends on the origin of the tumor. Treatment of

---

*Wright, J. E.: Unpublished paper, delivered at meeting of American Academy of Ophthalmology and Otolaryngology, Las Vegas, October 7, 1976.
†Henderson, J. W., and Neault, R. W.: En bloc removal of intrinsic neoplasms of the lacrymal gland. *Trans. of A.O.S.* 74:133, 1976.

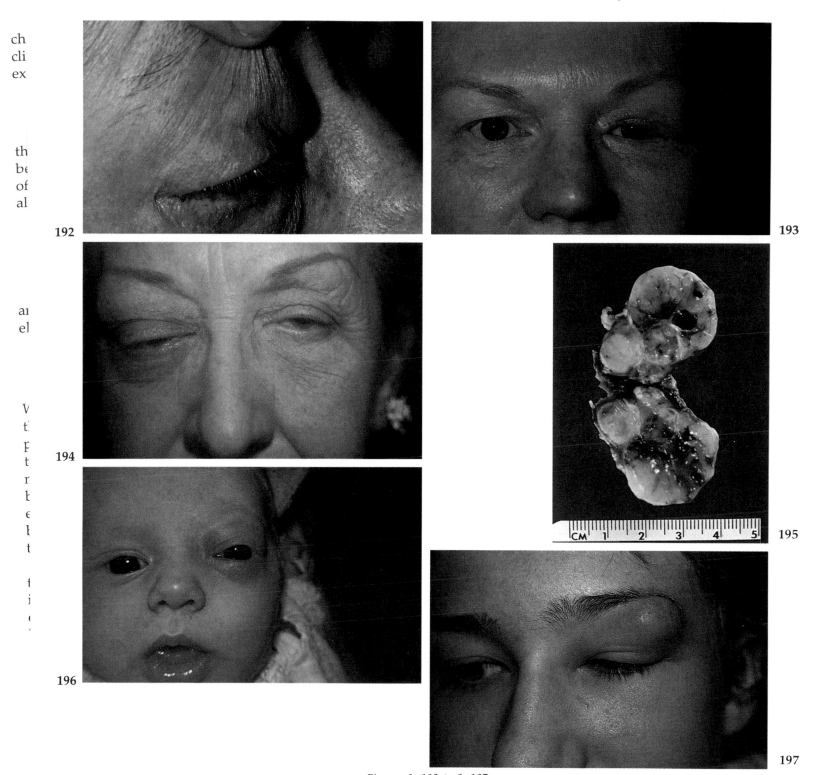

Figures 9–192 to 9–197

Figure 9–192 Lid mass represents part of lymphomatous process that involves lids, orbit, and scalp.

Figure 9–193 Forty-two year old woman with sudden onset of tender supratemporal mass. Vision 20/20. Biopsy revealed pseudotumor.

Figure 9–194 Fifty-five year old woman with history of a slow-growing (2 or 3 years) mass of superior temporal aspect of the right orbit. Excisional biopsy revealed mixed tumor of the lacrimal gland as shown in figure 9–195.

Figure 9–196 Orbital cellulitis.

Figure 9–197 Metastatic orbital abscess from infected blister on the heel.

297

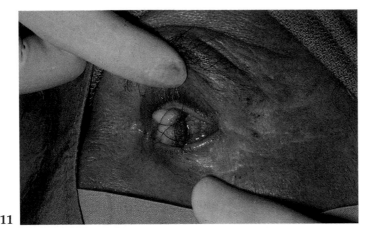

211

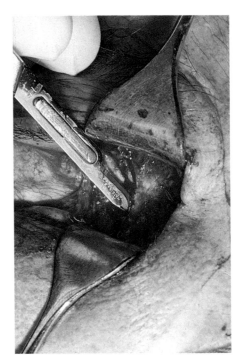

212

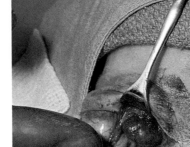

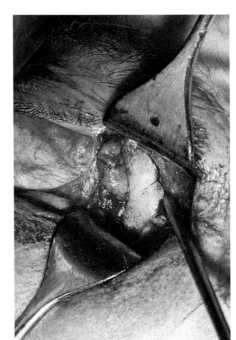

213

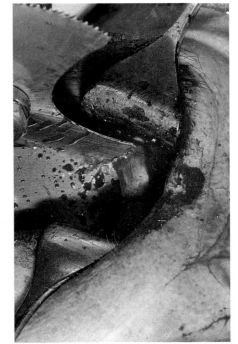

214   215

Fi
F:
F:
n
q
F
r
t
s

Figures 9–211 to 9–215

Figure 9–211 The cornea is protected with Gelfoam.

Figure 9–212 The periosteum is incised along the orbital rim.

Figure 9–213 The index finger is inserted between the bone and the periosteum as diagramed in figure 9–217. If the tumor is small and anteriorly located as the one indicated here it is not necessary to remove the lateral orbital wall.

Figure 9–214 If the wall is to be removed the periosteum is stripped from the orbital aspect of the rim and back into the temporal fossa.

Figure 9–215 The rim is cut with the Stryker saw.

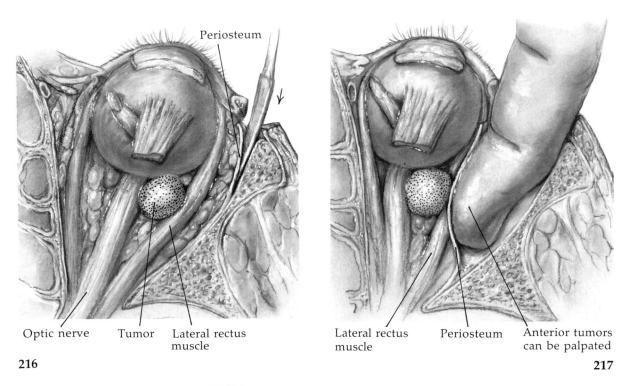

Periosteum

Optic nerve   Tumor   Lateral rectus
muscle

216

Lateral rectus   Periosteum   Anterior tumors
muscle   can be palpated

217

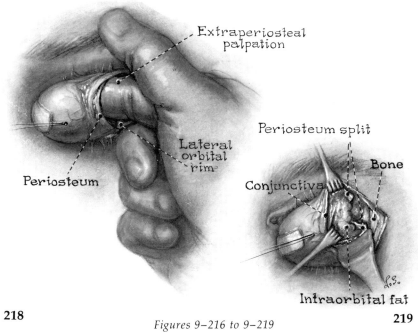

Extraperiosteal
palpation

Periosteum

Lateral
orbital
rim

Periosteum split

Bone

Conjunctiva

Intraorbital fat

218

Figures 9–216 to 9–219

219

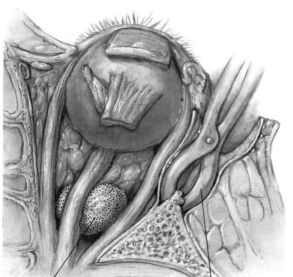

Figure 9–220

Tumor   Removing lateral
orbital wall

The thin lateral wall (zygomatic bone, Fig. 9–221) behind the heavy rim is removed with rongeurs as far back as the junction of the posterior orbital wall (orbital plate of the greater wing of the sphenoid bone) with the lateral wall (temporal bone) of the skull (Fig. 9–220). Bone bleeding may be encountered in the spongy bone at this depth and can be controlled with bone wax. The bone wax is softened, placed on the convex surface of the curved Freer elevator, and pushed firmly into the bleeding area. The excess wax is then removed.

The whole lateral half of the orbital contents is now exposed. The periosteum is intact but is usually quite pliable so that palpation can be done without difficulty (Figs. 9–222 and 9–223). An anteroposterior incision through the periosteum and periorbita is carefully done with Wescott scissors. All bleeding points are controlled. Fat usually prolapses into the incision and makes visualization difficult; it must be carefully retracted with spoon or flat retractors because vessels in the fat are unsupported and easily rupture, producing a deep hemorrhage that is hard to control. Palpation of the whole orbit can be done with the exception of the very nasal portion, making it possible to determine where the mass lies in relation to the muscle cone. If the tumor is in the muscle cone, the lateral rectus muscle is detached after a 5–0 catgut locking suture has been placed at its insertion. The muscle stump and the small bleeders of the globe are cauterized. A 4–0 black silk suture is placed at the site of the muscle insertion to act as a traction suture.

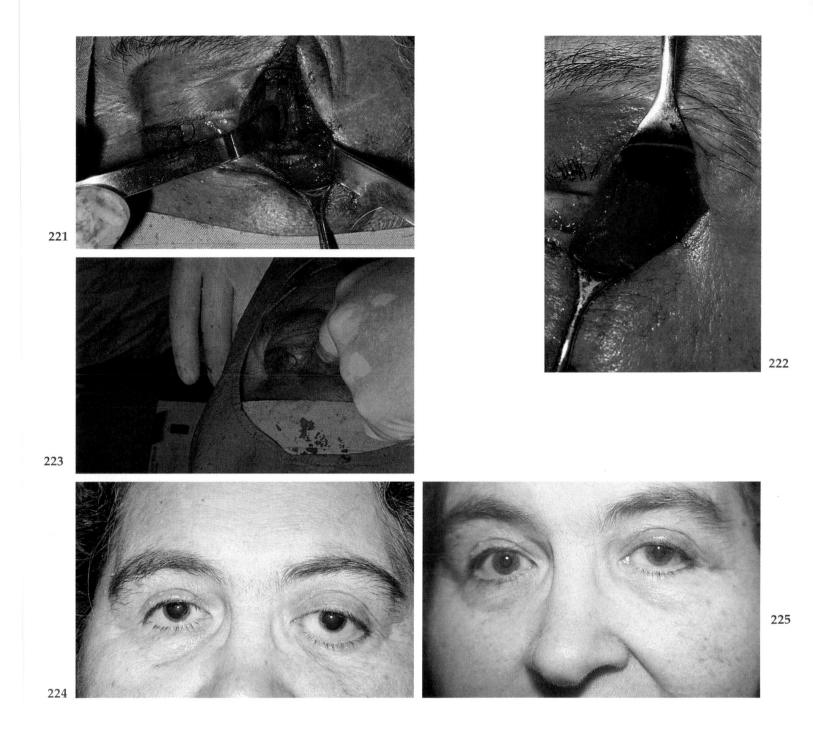

221

222

223

224

225

Figures 9–221 to 9–225

Figure 9–221 Orbital and temporal tissues are shown here retracted away from the thin lateral wall.

Figures 9–222 and 9–223 Palpation can be carried out through the periosteum.

Figure 9–224 Six month history of increasing left proptosis and decreasing vision to 20/50.

Figure 9–225 The patient pictured in figure 9–224 two months postoperatively removal of orbital hemangioma. Vision returned to 20/20.

Frontal Approach

NASAL BROW APPROACH

A nasal brow approach is used in removing primary tumors in the nasal orbit. (It is also used for removing mucoceles described in Chapter 7.) A curved incision is made just below the hair line of the nasal portion of the eyebrow and is carried down to the periosteum. It is preferable to stay nasal and behind the exit notch of the frontal nerve and vessels. At times, this is impossible; bleeding is then quite marked but can be controlled with cautery. Cutting the nerve causes anesthesia of the brow that may last for many months. The periosteum along the orbital rim is incised, and the trochlea is cut free from the bone by sharp dissection. The trochlea then can be separated with the periosteum as it is stripped from the bone as far posteriorly as is required for good exposure. The nasal orbit can be explored digitally and then visualized by retracting the contents laterally. The tumor is located, and an incision is made in the periosteum directly over it. The mass is delivered as is described for the lateral approach.

Closure consists of merely allowing the orbital contents to settle back into place. The periosteum and trochlea reattach themselves to the bony orbital wall without suturing. The brow incision is closed with 8–0 silk.

A combined lateral orbitotomy and frontal or nasal approach is often used. The lateral orbitotomy is added to give room to displace the eye temporally so a nasally placed tumor can be better exposed. This is particularly useful for tumors located in the nasal muscle cone.

LATERAL BROW APPROACH

A lateral brow approach (Figs. 9–227 and 9–228) is made for superficial tumors, chiefly dermoids at the orbital rim. The incision is made directly over the mass, through skin and subcutaneous tissue just beneath the hair line of the brow. If necessary, it can be enlarged laterally as far as the canthus and the ligament can be detached with the periosteum to give greater exposure. If this is done, periosteum and attached canthal ligament are resutured at the end of the procedure.

INFERIOR ANTERIOR APPROACH

The inferior anterior approach either nasally or temporally is usually used only for removing very superficial tumors or taking a biopsy.

CONJUNCTIVAL APPROACH

The conjuntival approach is rarely used for orbital tumors, with the exception of taking a biopsy or removing a superficial lymphoma for diagnosis.

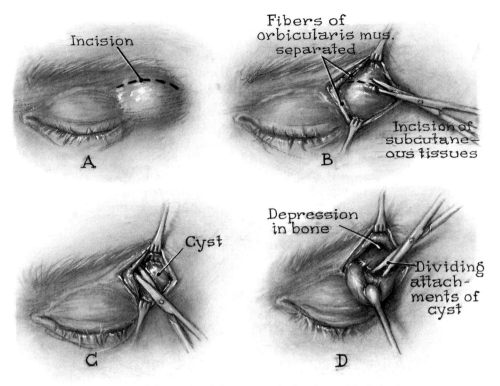

Figure 9–227   Schematic of the removal of a dermoid of the brow.

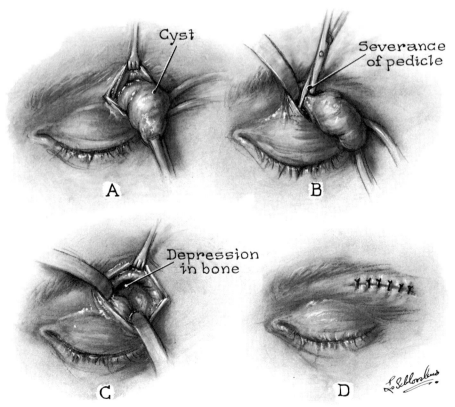

Figure 9–228   There is often a depression in the bone at the site of the dermoid. The cyst must be carefully removed by blunt and sharp dissection and cautery from the many fine fibrous attachments. *Great care is taken to avoid rupturing the sac.* A cryoprobe is helpful for traction on the mass.

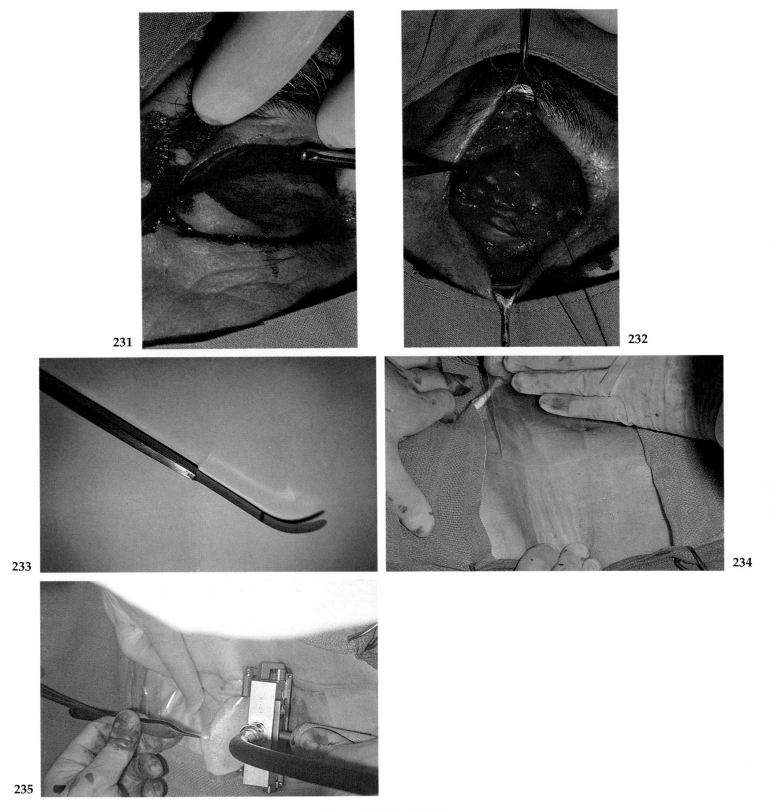

Figures 9–231 to 9–235

Figure 9–231 Incision is carried down to the bone along the orbital rim.
Figure 9–232 The periosteum is stripped from the orbital wall.
Figure 9–233 Exenteration knife.
Figure 9–234 Dermatome adhesive tape is applied firmly and smoothly.
Figure 9–235 The assistant supports the graft as it emerges from the dermatome.

This procedure leaves the orbital contents free from the bone except along the superior and inferior orbital fissures and at the apex. These areas are cut free from the bone by a specially designed exenteration knife (Iliff-Storz) (Fig. 9–233) which is directed along the temporal orbital wall between the bone and periosteum and advanced with a sweeping motion. If this exenteration knife is not available, curved enucleation scissors can be used, although with scissors it is impossible to remove the entire apical stump. The orbital contents are removed (Fig. 9–230), the orbit is immediately packed with dry gauze, and pressure is applied to control bleeding.

Pressure must be maintained by an assistant while the skin graft is being prepared. A 0.010 to 0.020 inch thick skin graft, 2 inches wide by 4 inches long, is cut from a hairless area of the inner surface of the thigh or from the abdomen. The Stryker dermatome, with a rapidly oscillating blade, is ideal for cutting the graft the desired thickness, but any dermatome can be used. A sterile, clear plastic adhesive tape (Stryker dermatome adhesive tape) is placed on the stretched skin (Fig. 9–234) to insure good contact with the blade and to prevent the skin from curling into a small ribbon. The gauge of the dermatome is set to compensate for the thickness of the plastic (the Stryker dermatome is calibrated to account for the adhesive thickness) and the dermatome is applied over the plastic and directed away from the surgeon since the graft presents itself in a strip ahead of the knife (Fig. 9–235). The dermatome must be applied with firm pressure: otherwise the graft may be irregular and tattered. The donor site is dressed with Vaseline (petrolatum) gauze and a firm pressure bandage. The importance of a smooth, thin graft cannot be overemphasized. A thick graft does not take well. Only the cells in contact with bone remain viable, so that superficial layers of a thick graft slough, leaving necrotic folds that are a nidus for infection.

The gauze pack is removed from the orbit (Fig. 9–238). Any slight ooze from the bone is controlled with wax. The apical stump should be heavily fulgurated to insure destruction of all tumor tissue and to completely control bleeding.

The skin graft (Figs. 9–236 and 9–239) is now shaped into a cone that fits into the orbit. The plastic tape facilitates handling and shaping of the thin graft; it must not be removed until the graft has been rolled into a cone and its overlapping sides have been cut and stitched together with fine silk sutures. After the cone is shaped and the sides are joined, the skin graft is peeled from the plastic. The anterior edge of the cone is carefully sutured to the skin of the orbital rim with 7–0 chromic catgut or 8–0 silk sutures that are placed about 3 mm apart (Fig. 9–240). The conical graft is pressed back into the orbit so as to cover everything but the apex.

Several stab holes are placed in the graft over the area of the superior and inferior orbital fissures to facilitate drainage, and the small end of the cone is left open to provide adequate drainage from the fulgurated area at the orbital apex. If the apex is covered, trapped drainage may lift the graft. This area will ultimately be epithelialized from proliferation of cells from the edge of the graft. Holding a gauze sponge against the apex with a hemostat discourages any slight apical ooze until the final sea sponge pack has been put in place. A thin conical layer of sterile sea sponge, shaped exactly like the graft (Fig. 9–237), is placed in the socket (Fig. 9–241)

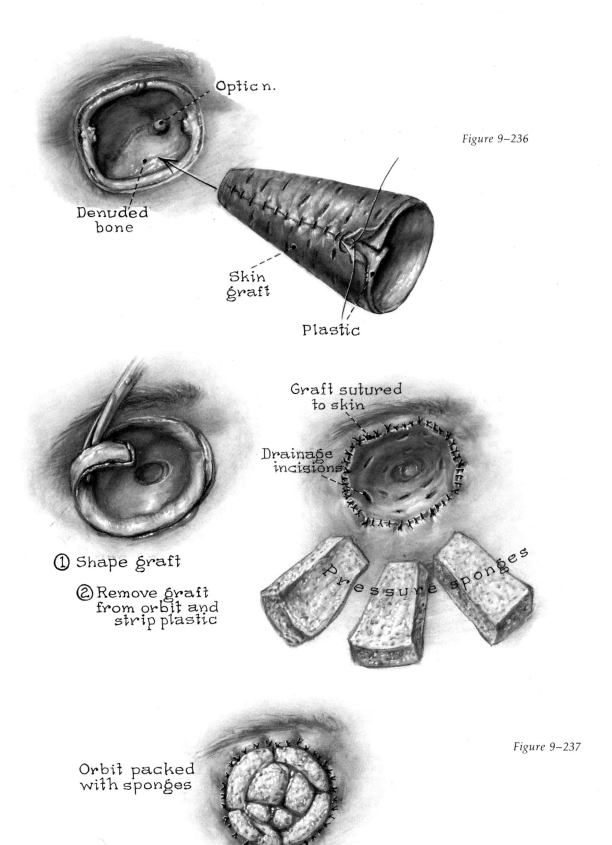

Optic n.

Denuded
bone

Skin
graft

Plastic

Figure 9–236

① Shape graft

② Remove graft
from orbit and
strip plastic

Graft sutured
to skin

Drainage
incisions

Pressure sponges

Orbit packed
with sponges

Figure 9–237

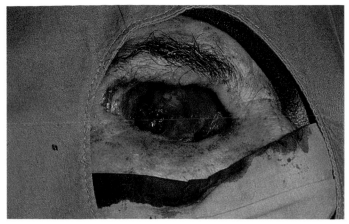

238

Figure 9–238   The orbit must be dry prior to insertion of the graft.
Figure 9–239   The graft is rolled into a cone.
Figure 9–240   An extremely thin graft can easily be stretched to fill the orbit.
Figure 9–241   The sea sponges are inserted in layers.
Figure 9–242   Postoperative exenteration.
Figure 9–243   Patient pictured in figure 9–242 with prosthesis fitted.

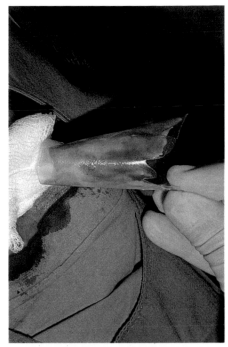

239

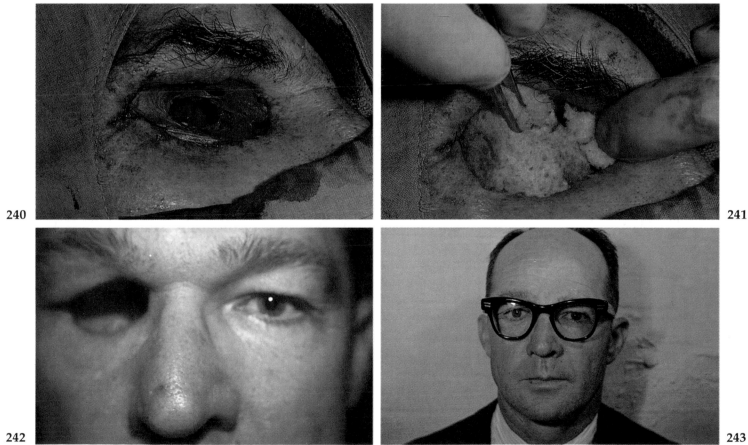

240

241

242

243

Figures 9–238 to 9–243

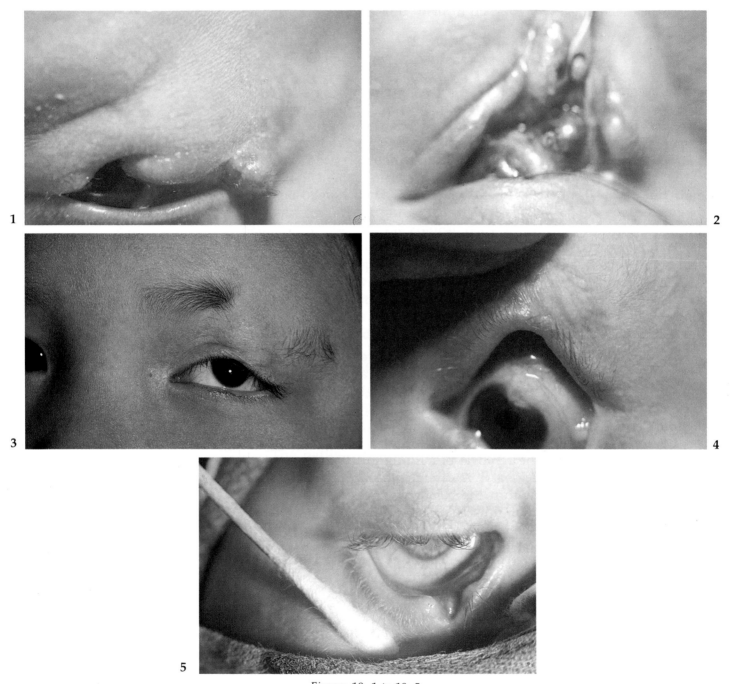

Figures 10–1 to 10–5

Figure 10–1 Upper lid coloboma.

Figure 10–2 Elevation of lid of patient in figure 10–1 reveals staphyloma of the globe.

Figures 10–3 and 10–4 The appearance several years postoperative repair of the coloboma pictured in 10–1. Essentially normal lid margin.

Figure 10–5 Lower lid coloboma.

no surgery should be done unless the condition persists after puberty. On the other hand, there are some patients in whom the epicanthus (with associated blepharophimosis) is severe. A heavy epicanthal fold produces the misleading appearance of an esotropia because of a complete coverage of the inner canthal structures. Z- and Y-V-plasty procedures have been suggested, but the skin and subcutaneous tissues in these children is thickened and scars following surgery fade slowly.

No perfect solution seems to be at hand, but Mustardé* has given the most recent spur to the surgical endeavors. He has described a procedure whereby triangular skin flaps are transposed in such a way that the vertical distance in the area of the fold is increased and the horizontal decreased. This relieves the vertical tension that has produced the fold. The medial canthus is then pulled nasally by shortening the medial canthal ligament.

A horizontal cut is made with scissors through the epicanthal fold overlying the medial canthus. Depending on the extent of the fold, this cut will be 10 to 15 mm long when traction is placed on the medial end (A-C) (Fig. 10–6). Paramarginal incisions are extended from the temporal end (C) of the incision along the upper and lower lids for 8 to 10 mm (C-D) (Fig. 10–7). The area above and below is undermined for approximately 1 cm.

An incision of 8 mm is extended superotemporally and inferotemporally at an angle of 60 degrees from the midpoint of A-C (B) to a point E. From E, at an angle of 45 degrees to B-E, an incision is directed nasally for about 8 mm to F (Figs. 10–8 and 10–9). The medial canthal ligament is exposed and either an imbrication of the ligament or a resection is done to move the inner canthus nasally as far as desired. We have used 4–0 siliconized silk sutures for this.

The shaded areas B-D are then trimmed to facilitate proper fit of the flaps to be rotated (Fig. 10–9). The triangles B-E-F and E-B-D are then transposed (B' to F and E' to D) increasing the vertical dimension and decreasing the horizontal (Fig. 10–10). The skin is closed with 7–0 absorbable sutures (Fig. 10–11).

Telecanthus

A widening of the intercanthal distance may be familial (Figs. 10–12 and 10–13), and even the best of corrective procedures does not make these patients look normal. Correction consists primarily of shortening the medial canthal ligaments combined with, if necessary, a Z-plasty of the epicanthal area as has been described in the previous section. Lateral canthotomy is often necessary to provide proper size and centering of the palpebral fissure. If medial canthal shortening by itself will suffice, a small incision is made horizontally extending nasally from (but not including) the medial

*Mustardé, J. C.: Chapter 12. *In* Tessier, P., et al., *Symposium on Plastic Surgery in the Orbital Region.* Vol. 12, C. V. Mosby Co., St. Louis, 1976.

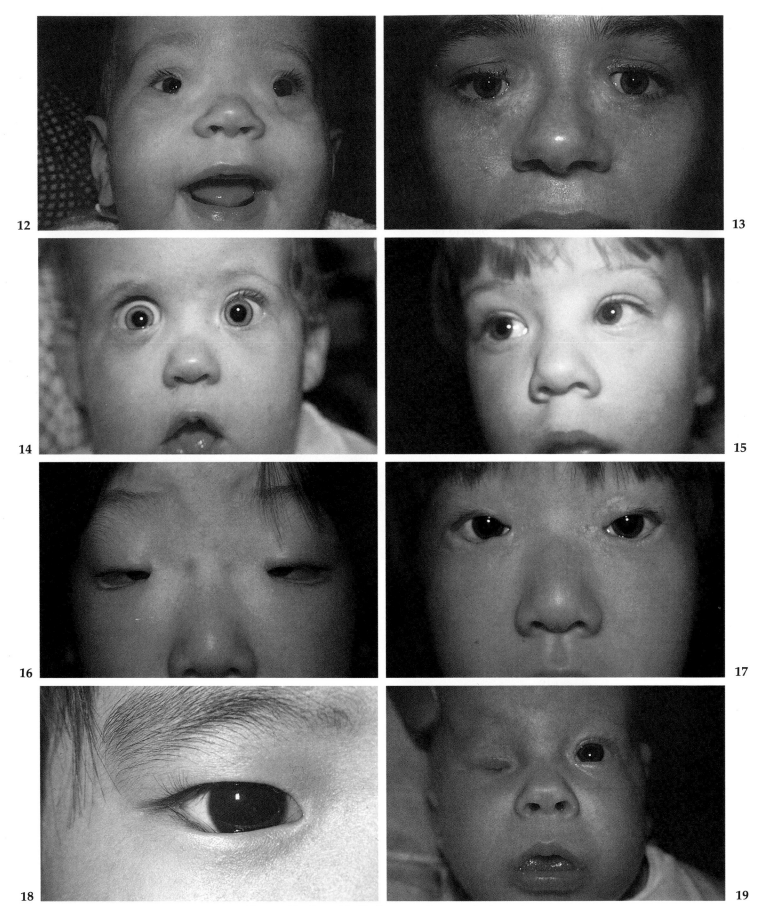

Figures 10–12 to 10–19. See opposite page for legend.

324

canthus. Retraction superiorly and inferiorly allows the blunt dissection and isolation of the medial canthal ligament. The ligament is then imbricated (usually as much as is possible) and sutured with a strong nonabsorbable suture such as 4–0 siliconized silk. If a lateral canthotomy is done, the raw edges are not sutured. Rather, bleeding is carefully stopped with cautery, and the area is left to epithelialize. Following the initial routine canthotomy incision, the lid margins may have to be trimmed to give proper contour. The canthotomy usually needs to be reopened daily for several days.

Transnasal wiring for the repair of congenital telecanthus has been suggested; however, we have not found it necessary to employ this technique.

Lid Retraction

Upper Lid

Upper lid retraction is usually associated with thyroid disease or neurological abnormality (Parinaud's syndrome, aberrant third nerve regeneration). Rarely, however, it does occur congenitally, associated with a fibrotic levator and superior rectus muscle (Fig. 10–14). Forced duction tests will demonstrate the restriction of motion of the superior rectus muscle. The levator should be lengthened by placing a scleral insert in the aponeurosis where it narrows to join the levator muscle (Fig. 10–15). (See lengthening of the levator in thyroid disease, p. 152.) The superior rectus should be recessed at a later date.

Lower Lid

Lower lid retraction, actually a ptosis and ectropion of the outer one half of the lid, occurs in some children with a congenital ptosis of the upper lids (frequently in association with blepharophimosis) (Fig. 10–16) but also is a common occurrence in the Treacher-Collins syndrome, with an associated defect of the malar bones and low or absent external ears. In these children, it is usually possible to increase the vertical height of the tarsus of the lower lid by a free transplant of tarsus and conjunctiva from the retrotarsal margin of the upper lid to the lower edge of the tarsus of the lower lid. The method for obtaining a tarsal conjunctival graft from the retrotarsal margin is discussed under entropion of the upper lid (p. 141). A

Figure 10–12   Marked telecanthus.

Figure 10–13   Mother of patient in figure in 10–12 had corrective surgery as a child.

Figure 10–14   Right upper lid retraction.

Figure 10–15   Five years postoperative repair of right upper lid retraction pictured in figure 10–14.

Figure 10–16   Ptosis of the lower lids may be a minor aspect of the presentation but may be quite glaring following correction of telecanthus and ptosis of the upper lids.

Figure 10–17   Patient in figure 10–16 after Mustardé procedure for telecanthus, bilateral frontalis slings, and elevation of the lower lids using tarsus excised from the upper lids.

Figure 10–18   Epiblepharon.

Figure 10–19   Anophthalmus.

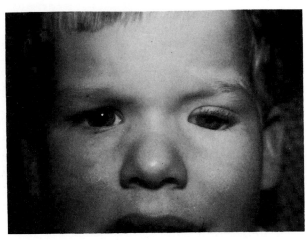

Figure 10–20   Five years postoperative picture of the patient depicted in figure 10–19. Normal orbit growth has been achieved.

skin and muscle flap from above the upper lid crease is rotated down to increase the vertical height of the anterior portion of the lower lid. The upper lid is elevated somewhat as a result of the shortening of tarsus and removal of skin (Fig. 10–17).

EPIBLEPHARON

Epiblepharon consists of an extra fold of skin that runs across the lid close to the lid margin and because of its tightness turns the lashes against the cornea (Fig. 10–18). Most of these relax after the first year of life, so surgery should be delayed unless corneal abrasion occurs.

Should surgery be indicated, the tightened horizontal fold of skin and pretarsal muscle can be removed by an elliptical incision. Care should be taken to remove only the excess tightened skin so that when the incision edges are reapproximated, lashes evert to the normal position. Excision of too much skin and orbicularis will cause ectropion. In rare cases Z-plasty, particularly at the medial canthus, is necessary to relieve excessive horizontal skin tension. It must be remembered, however, that because the skin and subcutaneous tissues in these children are somewhat thick, scars are often hard to hide and may be prominent for several years. Incisions should always be oriented with natural skin lines, but this may be difficult to do in these children. The sutures described for spastic or involutional entropion will not work for this congenital condition.

Anophthalmos

The globe may be absent (Fig. 10–19) or a small nubbin of an eye may be present. To stimulate the normal growth of the bony orbit and to improve the cosmetic appearance, a prosthesis is placed in the area of the muscle cone. As the child grows, the prosthesis is replaced by a larger one every 3 to 4 years. We have found inflatable silicone implants (American Optical Company) to be especially useful as they can be inserted in collapsed form through a small incision in the center of the conjunctiva and then reinflated. Often a small deformed or cystic globe is present, which is removed when the implant is inserted. In order to avoid the abnormal firm fibrous tissue that is sometimes present, particularly peripherally in the orbit, the incision should be made in the center of the conjunctiva (or in the area of the abnormal or cystic globe). Closure of Tenon's capsule and conjunctiva is done in separate layers, using absorbable interrupted sutures. A prosthesis is inserted to prevent cul-de-sac contracture (Fig. 10–20).

Lacrimal Tract

Absent or occluded puncta, congenital fistulas, and occlusion of the inferior end of the lacrimal tract are discussed under lacrimal surgery (p. 186).

Cilia Abnormalities

Distichiasis consists of an accessory row of lashes, which often present through or behind the orifices of the meibomian glands. If the lashes are relatively sparse they can be removed by electrolysis. If this is not successful, a strip of the posterior edge of the lid containing the aberrant lashes is removed, and the defect is filled with a strip of tarsus and conjunctiva from the retrotarsal margin, as described for entropion of the upper lid (p. 141).

11
Trauma

Lacerations

Reconstruction of the lids or orbit after trauma demands a flexible approach; preliminary plans may need to be altered as the surgeon proceeds with the repair. Thus, a teacher should confine his advice to the basic principles unless he can be at the operative scene. Of first importance is the globe, and lacerations of the lid or fractures of the orbit must not be permitted to mask injury to the eye.

Deep lacerations of the lids should be repaired under general anesthesia; each structure must be identified and replaced as nearly as possible in its anatomical position. Because of the general condition of the patient, immediate repair of the adnexal injury may not be practical. In such cases, a moist antibiotic pack on the lids helps keep the tissues pliable, while passage of time allows for the reduction of edema.

We agree with Mustardé* that the repair of the tarsus is the most important single factor in effecting an acceptable functional and cosmetic result. A lacerated lid will heal with the least disfigurement if the cut tarsal edges are accurately approximated with small buried stitches of fine suture material (Figs. 11–1 and 11–2). This is at variance with the writings of some early ophthalmic surgeons who advocated halving techniques or the splitting or step methods. Such techniques, beautifully presented by the medical illustrators, look better on the printed page than in the operating room, and to some extent, waste lid tissue that may be necessary for reconstruction.

Great care should be taken to obtain all severed tissue, as skin or even whole lids that have been severed for several hours may remain viable (Figs. 11–3 to 11–9). The current practice is careful conservation of tissue and replacement of lost tissue with like tissue. There has been a fortunate shift away from using the forehead or cheek flaps for secondary repair, as that skin is thick and does

---

*Mustardé, J.: Address given at New York Academy of Ophthalmology, 1971.

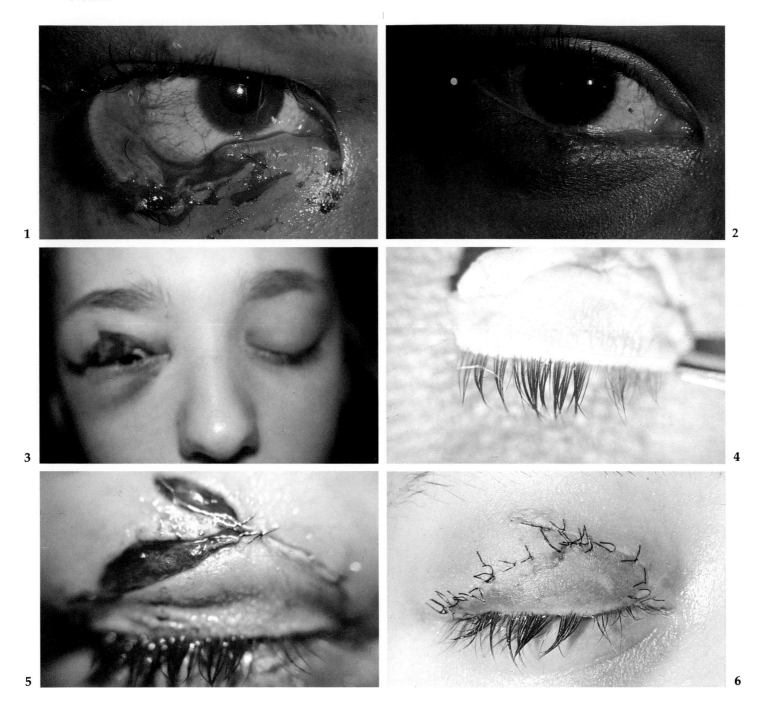

Figures 11–1 to 11–6

Figure 11–1 Ragged tarsal laceration, the result of a human bite. Repair consisted of careful reapproximation of tissues, with no trimming of laceration margins. Tarsal layer was closed with 6–0 chromic catgut, and lid margin and skin reapproximated with 8–0 silk.

Figure 11–2 Appearance of patient in Figure 11–1, three weeks postoperatively.

Figure 11–3 Complete avulsion of 80 per cent of the upper lid secondary to horse bite.

Figure 11–4 Severed lid recovered from stable floor 5 hours later.

Figure 11–5 Severed piece sutured in place.

Figure 11–6 Healing of sutured piece.

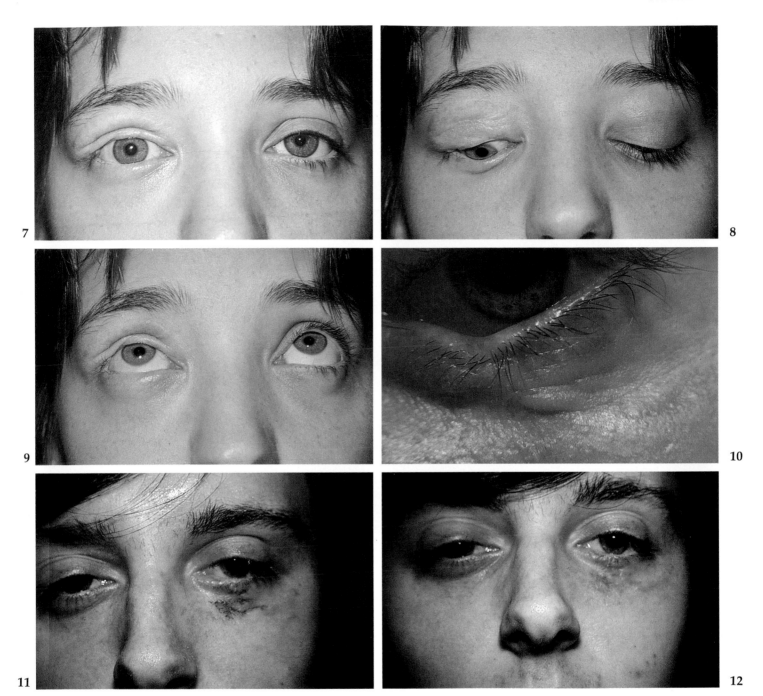

Figures 11–7 to 11–12

Figures 11–7 to 11–9 Postoperatively, good lid contour and function. The result is superior to what might have been possible if the severed piece had not been used. The lashes that were lost can best be replaced with glued-on cosmetic lashes.

Figure 11–10 Patient with scarring and lid notching following laceration repair.

Figure 11–11 Immediately postoperative excision of scar and Z-plasty done to relieve the lid notching due to vertical shortening caused by the scar.

Figure 11–12 Two weeks after removal of sutures.

not give the functional and cosmetic results that tissue from a fellow lid can give.

Lacerations from glass or a sharp instrument may be of any configuration, depth, or extent. Careful approximation of the cut edges with very fine suture material will reduce scarring in this lax, soft tissue. If a lid has been improperly repaired as a primary procedure, the wound should be reopened and the edges freshened and repaired properly. If scarring has occurred, it must be excised or relaxed (Figs. 11–10 to 11–12).

A tearing laceration by a hook, a tooth, or a finger ruptures the lid at its weakest point (Figs. 11–13 to 11–15), i.e., near the inner canthus, where the tarsus ends and the upper and lower canthal ligaments are at their thinnest. The tear usually extends vertically across the canaliculus and as far as the orbital rim and then horizontally. If only one canaliculus is damaged, the fellow uninjured canaliculus in its normal state will allow adequate drainage of tears; therefore, the surgeon should avoid disturbing the uninjured tract with probes or similar instruments.

The canaliculus may be lacerated near the punctum in its relatively horizontal course; here the cut ends of the tract can usually be easily located and a Viers stainless steel rod (Davis and Geck) inserted to splint the canaliculus during the healing period. The stent consists of a small steel rod with a silk suture swaged to one end. The rod is positioned in the cut tract, and the cut edges of the canaliculus are approximated under the microscope, using 9–0 or 10–0 nylon. Conjunctiva and skin are closed in the usual fashion and provide additional support. The swaged silk suture extending out through the punctum is sutured to the skin to prevent migration of the rod deep into the sac.

If a Viers rod is not available, several procedures are possible. Byron Smith has made a splint by using a 2–0 black silk suture swaged to a round needle, cutting off the sharp point of the needle and straightening it. He reports this works very well. We have used a 0.025 inch Silastic tube (not polyethylene) threaded through the punctum into the sac (Fig. 11–16), using a No. 00 Bowman probe as a stylet. The Silastic tube is fastened to the lower cul-de-sac by 8–0 sutures in several spots. It slightly inverts the punctum, but lying in this position, it causes no trauma to the cornea. Bennett uses No. 1 chromic catgut for a stent, which he leaves in place 10 to 12 days.*

Deep lacerations that come close to the common canaliculus almost always scar severely and result in loss of function of the canaliculus. In these instances preservation of the undamaged tract is of primary importance. For this reason, tubes that loop or circle through both tracts and are pulled down into the nose are not recommended because of the potential trauma to the uninjured tract during insertion.

However, when the upper and lower canaliculi and the canthal ligament all have been damaged, a loop of Silastic threaded through both puncta and brought out into the sac or even carried down into

---

*Bennett, J. E.: Lacrimal Drainage System. *In*: *Clinical Ophthalmology*. Harper and Row, Hagerstown, Md., 1976.

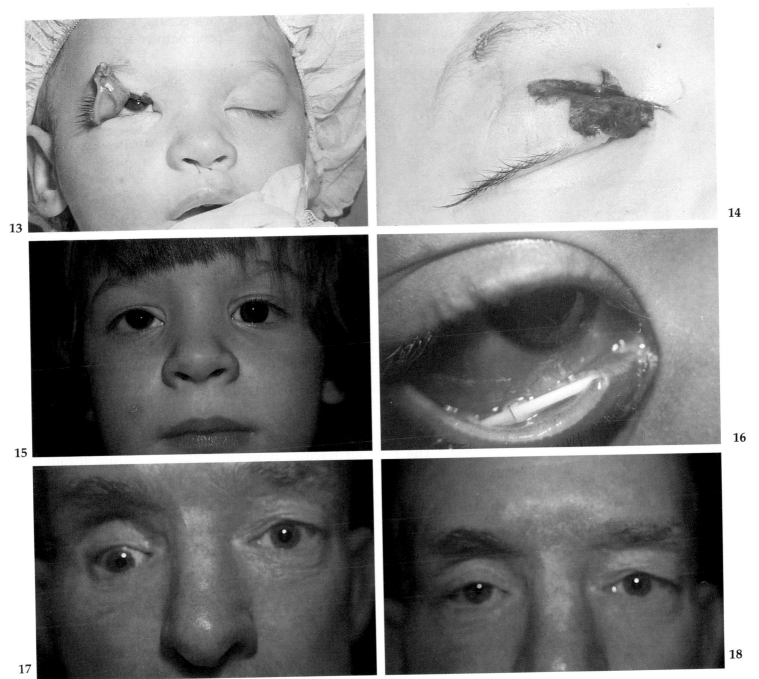

13
14
15
16
17
18

Figures 11–13 to 11–18

Figure 11–13   Laceration resulting from patient's falling on a display board hook.

Figure 11–14   The lid is returned to the proper anatomical position.

Figure 11–15   The patient in figure 11–14 and 11–15 three years postoperatively.

Figure 11–16   Canaliculus kept open with Silastic tube sutured into the inferior cul-de-sac.

Figures 11–17 and 11–18   Pre and postoperative repair of orbital floor fracture which had caused enophthalmos and left hypertropia.

Index

Note: *Italicized* numbers indicate illustrations.